Drug Safety: Managing Innovation in Rheumatology

Editors

JOHN J. CUSH
KATHRYN H. DAO

RHEUMATIC DISEASE CLINICS OF NORTH AMERICA

www.rheumatic.theclinics.com

November 2012 • Volume 38 • Number 4

ELSEVIER

1600 John F. Kennedy Blvd., Suite 1800 ● Philadelphia, PA 19103-2899
http://www.theclinics.com

RHEUMATIC DISEASE CLINICS OF NORTH AMERICA Volume 38, Number 4
November 2012 ISSN 0889-857X, ISBN 13: 978-1-4557-5065-8

Editor: Pamela Hetherington

Rheumatic Disease Clinics of North America (ISSN 0889-857X) is published quarterly by Elsevier Inc., 360 Park Avenue South, New York, NY 10010-1710. Months of issue are February, May, August, and November. Business and editorial offices: 1600 John F. Kennedy Boulevard, Suite 1800, Philadelphia, PA 19103-2899. Periodicals postage paid at New York, NY and additional mailing offices. Subscription prices are USD 305.00 per year for US individuals, USD 534.00 per year for US institutions, USD 150.00 per year for US students and residents, USD 360.00 per year for Canadian individuals, USD 659.00 per year for Canadian institutions, USD 427.00 per year for international individuals, USD 659.00 per year for international institutions, and USD 210.00 per year for Canadian and foreign students/residents. To receive student/resident rate, orders must be accompanied by name of affiliated institution, date of term, and the *signature* of program/residency coordinator on institution letterhead. Orders will be billed at individual rate until proof of status received. Foreign air speed delivery is included in all *Clinics* subscription prices. All prices are subject to change without notice. **POSTMASTER:** Send address changes to *Rheumatic Disease Clinics of North America,* Elsevier Health Sciences Division, Subscription Customer Service, 3251 Riverport Lane, Maryland Heights, MO 63043. **Customer Service: 1-800-654-2452 (US and Canada). From outside of the US and Canada: 314-447-8871. Fax: 314-447-8029. For print support, e-mail: JournalsCustomerService-usa@elsevier.com. For online support, e-mail: JournalsOnline Support-usa@elsevier.com.**

Reprints. For copies of 100 or more of articles in this publication, please contact the Commercial Reprints Department, Elsevier Inc., 360 Park Avenue South, New York, New York, 10010-1710; Tel.: (+1) 212-633-3813, Fax: (+1) 212-462-1935, and E-mail: reprints@elsevier.com.

Rheumatic Disease Clinics of North America is covered in *MEDLINE/PubMed (Index Medicus), Current Contents/Clinical Medicine, Science Citation Index, ISI/BIOMED,* and *EMBASE/Excerpta Medica.*

Printed and bound by CPI Group (UK) Ltd, Croydon, CR0 4YY

Transferred to digital print 2012

Contributors

CONSULTING EDITOR

MICHAEL H. WEISMAN, MD
Director, Division of Rheumatology; Professor of Medicine, Cedars-Sinai Medical Center, Los Angeles, California

GUEST EDITORS

JOHN J. CUSH, MD
Director of Clinical Rheumatology, Baylor Research Institute; Professor of Medicine and Rheumatology, Baylor University Medical Center, Dallas, Texas

KATHRYN H. DAO, MD
Associate Director of Rheumatology Research, Baylor Research Institute, Dallas, Texas

AUTHORS

JOHN J. CUSH, MD
Director of Clinical Rheumatology, Baylor Research Institute; Professor of Medicine and Rheumatology, Baylor University Medical Center, Dallas, Texas

KATHRYN H. DAO, MD
Associate Director of Rheumatology Research, Baylor Research Institute, Dallas, Texas

RICHARD FURIE, MD
Professor of Medicine, Hofstra North Shore–Long Island Jewish School of Medicine; Chief, Division of Rheumatology and Allergy-Clinical Immunology, North Shore–Long Island Jewish Health System, Lake Success, New York

SUSAN M. GOODMAN, MD
Division of Rheumatology, Hospital For Special Surgery, New York, New York

NADIA HABAL, MD
Northern Virginia Arthritis, Alexandria, Virginia

MORLEY HERBERT, PhD
Medical City Dallas Hospital, Dallas, Texas

ROBERT T. KEENAN, MD, MPH
Assistant Professor of Medicine; Director, Duke Gout and Crystal Arthropathies Clinic; Medical Director, Duke Specialty Infusion Center; Division of Rheumatology and Immunology, Department of Medicine, Duke University School of Medicine, Durham, North Carolina

NAIM M. MAALOUF, MD
Assistant Professor of Medicine, Department of Internal Medicine, Center for Mineral Metabolism and Clinical Research, University of Texas Southwestern Medical Center, Dallas, Texas

ASHIMA MAKOL, MD
Division of Rheumatology, Mayo Clinic College of Medicine, Rochester, Minnesota

RICHARD W. MARTIN, MD, MA
Professor of Medicine, Rheumatology, College of Human Medicine, Michigan State University, Grand Rapids, Michigan

ERIC L. MATTESON, MD, MPH
Division of Rheumatology, Mayo Clinic College of Medicine, Rochester, Minnesota

JOSEPH MOSAK, MD
Fellow, Division of Rheumatology and Allergy-Clinical Immunology, North Shore–Long Island Jewish Health System, Lake Success, New York

CATALINA OROZCO, MD
Rheumatology Associates, Dallas, Texas

STEPHEN PAGET, MD
Physician-in-Chief Emeritus, Division of Rheumatology, Hospital For Special Surgery; Professor of Medicine, Internal Medicine, Weill Cornell Medical College, New York, New York

KEVIN L. WINTHROP, MD, MPH
Associate Professor of Infectious Diseases, Public Health and Preventive Medicine, Oregon Health and Science University, Portland, Oregon

KERRY WRIGHT, MD
Division of Rheumatology, Mayo Clinic College of Medicine, Rochester, Minnesota

Contents

> When proposing a new therapy, rheumatologists must inform patients of a range of therapeutic options and support them towards making an informed decision. This article introduces definitions of equipoise and a good decision, contrasts persuasion from informed patient choice, and discussed the effects of patient characteristics including cognition on decision making. It also describes and offers examples of techniques and visual formats utilized in patient decision aids to present risk estimates to reduce cognitive bias and maximize patient comprehension.

> Gout is a metabolic disorder of purine metabolism and uric acid elimination. Over time, acute gout can develop into a chronic, disabling arthropathy, often associated with multiple comorbidities. Gout patients have often been undertreated, partly because of the clinician's perceived risks of a therapy outweighing its potential benefits. The approval of new therapies to treat hyperuricemia in gout has led to a new understanding of gout management and medication safety regarding new and old therapies. This review focuses on potential safety issues of currently available urate-lowering therapies and outlines strategies to minimize risks so their benefits can be reached.

> Bisphosphonates are antiresorptive medications widely prescribed for treating osteoporosis. In placebo-controlled clinical trials they have been shown to significantly reduce the risk of osteoporotic fractures. However, reports of atypical femoral fractures and osteonecrosis of the jaw have emerged with long-term use, raising questions regarding their long-term safety. Additionally, questions have also emerged regarding the association between bisphosphonates and other rare adverse events, such as esophageal cancer and atrial fibrillation. This article summarizes the current knowledge regarding the major side effects associated with the use of bisphosphonates, identifies at-risk populations for these side effects, and provides guidance for their use.

chronic conditions that predate or develop post-RA diagnosis. Increased mortality in RA is predominantly from nonarticular causes. The expanded armamentarium of disease-modifying drugs and biologics available has revolutionized management of articular disease but has made safe treatment of RA more complex. Drug-induced organ injury and side effects need to be kept in mind when initiating or modifying therapy.

Systemic lupus erythematosus (SLE) is the prototypic autoimmune disease with diverse clinical manifestations, affecting virtually all organ systems. A wide variety of medications are used for treatment, depending on organ involvement and severity. This article summarizes the adverse effects associated with different drugs currently used to treat SLE.

RHEUMATIC DISEASE CLINICS OF NORTH AMERICA

FORTHCOMING ISSUES

RECENT ISSUES

RELATED INTEREST

Hematology/Oncology Clinics of North America,
Volume 26, (October 2012)
http://www.hemonc.theclinics.com/current
Non-CML Myeloproliferative Diseases
Ross L. Levine, *Guest Editor*

NOW AVAILABLE FOR YOUR iPhone and iPad

Foreword

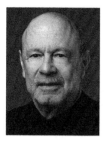

Michael H. Weisman, MD
Consulting Editor

This issue of *Rheumatic Disease Clinics of North America,* addresses one of the most significant issues facing the rheumatologist today—drug safety in a changing world where rheumatoid arthritis (RA) severity is less, patients are being identified and treated at a very early stage, and prevention is on the horizon. Are our drugs responsible for these events or are there secular trends behind the scenes causing these changing times? Regardless of the answer to this question, it is clear that our treatment decisions are going to be more and more based on the new horizons created by comorbidities and risk of aggressive treatments in vulnerable patients who may not even evolve into RA. This issue is dedicated to those issues.

Dao and colleagues demonstrate that the rate of nonserious infectious events is increased in biologic-treated subjects compared to standard DMARD therapies. This is revealed in a carefully performed meta-analysis of clinical trials with matched controls; the studies were almost all industry-sponsored with fairly similar definitions of the events in question. The monoclonal antibodies infliximab and adalimumab have a higher risk compared to etanercept, matching what is known about more serious infections including tuberculosis. What is not surprising based on our collective experience is that these infections tend to be self-limiting; however, we still are unsure if the anti-TNF drugs should be suspended when the nonserious infections such as URIs or flu symptoms actually occur on treatment.

Orozco and Maaloof carefully review the data on serious side effects linked to bisphosphonate use including osteonecrosis of the jaw and atypical femoral fractures; these risks are low and most importantly much less than the risks of fracture from untreated osteoporosis. Based on a risk-benefit analysis, they conclude that after 3 to 5 years one needs to reevaluate the need for continued bisphosphonate therapies in light of the need for continued benefit.

Makol, Wright, and Matteson clearly point out the challenges ahead in RA management by noting the complex array of comorbidities facing the clinician with the expanded armamentarium of agents that can affect almost all organ systems. Compared to the diseases themselves, these comorbidity issues may even have a greater impact on the safety of the drugs we typically employ.

Rheum Dis Clin N Am 38 (2012) ix–x
http://dx.doi.org/10.1016/j.rdc.2012.09.004
0889-857X/12/$ – see front matter

Richard Martin provides us with a critically important comment on drug safety—the patient's perspective. He points out that therapeutic decisions are made over time and typically involve multiple stakeholders especially when drugs have unique risks or sometimes when we are addressing a specific target population (ie, children/parental dyad). His article describes the characteristics of a sound decision that addresses patient characteristics to maximize comprehension with balanced information so that the physician can facilitate a good decision.

Kevin Winthrop, an infectious disease expert and an epidemiologist, faces the issue of serious infections in the biologic era, pointing out that RA itself increases the risk; on balance he feels the data addressing biologic therapies support some increase risk with these agents, typically in the first 6 to 12 months after a drug start. However, Winthrop addresses critical elements of a real-world practice that include prevention of infection in patients using biologics, including screening and vaccination, and the ever-important need to reduce the impact of harm caused by corticosteroids in our patients.

Robert Keenan notes that despite a new awakening of interest in gout and the advent of new therapies, the quality of care delivered to gout patients remains inadequate. He points out the complex interplay of major comorbidities in gout patients and our lack of appreciation of strategies that can be used to minimize risks of therapies. In the same vein, Mosak and Furie review the toxicities of drugs used to treat patients with systemic lupus erythematosus, emphasizing strategies to minimize these everpresent problems even with the most benign of our agents.

Goodman and Paget come to grips with an issue that is never standardized yet often addressed firmly and authoritatively without data—the perioperative management of the RA patient. They point out the balance needed between wound healing and infection risk versus needed disease control and postoperative rehabilitation that is critical for surgical outcome and control of health care costs. They give us answers where data are present as well as provide us with their experience in a health care setting where more of these decisions are made every day compared to where most of us work.

Cush analyzes a major issue facing treating rheumatologists today—do biologic agents increase the risk for malignancy beyond the risk associated with the disease itself? What do the data tell us about overall cancer risk, solid tumors risk alone, or risk of the most common malignancy in RA—lymphoma? Is cancer recurrence increased with biologics? Finally, if a cancer occurs on a biologic, is it more serious and what do you do with the biologic? Dr Cush goes as far as the data take him and then gives his most informed opinion.

Michael H. Weisman, MD
Division of Rheumatology
Cedars-Sinai Medical Center
8700 Beverly Boulevard
Los Angeles, CA 90024, USA

E-mail address:
michael.weisman@cshs.org

Preface

Refining Drug Safety in Rheumatology

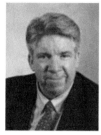 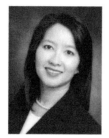

John J. Cush, MD   Kathryn H. Dao, MD
Guest Editors

An exciting era of rheumatology is upon us. Advances in pathobiology have produced novel advances in the treatment of rheumatoid arthritis, osteoarthritis, osteoporosis, gout, and lupus, to name a few. New and emerging therapeutics have substantially helped control symptoms and may also alter the natural history of progression and allow a chance for remission. Paradigm shifts in therapeutics are often a consequence of both novel drug development and wiser or more efficient use of existing therapies. While new treatment choices may be welcomed, they may also incite concern and caution. In this issue of *Rheumatic Disease Clinics of North America* we shed light on a variety of drug safety issues germane to the practice of rheumatology.

The need for change is driven by the lack of preventative or curative measures, clinical trial evidence of limited efficacy, and the ever-present practice of cycling patients through numerous therapies—either because of lack of efficacy, tolerability, or finances. It is not surprising that patients and physicians alike express enthusiasm over new treatments—as these may be "the magic bullet" we seek.

However, enthusiasm is ultimately trumped by concerns whether any agent "is truly safe." Pisetsky and others have stated that the safest risk is the one not taken.[1] During training, young doctors are taught by their mentors that therapeutic adventurism should be avoided. Rather than prescribe the "latest and greatest" new drug, the wise clinician should let others and time establish the safety of these novel therapies.[2] Hence while large controlled studies have shown significant clinical and radiographic benefits with new biologic agents in rheumatoid arthritis, the uptake of these agents by prescribers has been predictably slow. This change delay has been shown in many medical disciplines. Despite evidence favoring the cardioprotective effects of beta-blockers, lipid-lowering agents, and low-dose aspirin, the uptake of these in routine practice has also been disappointedly slow.[3] Perhaps clinicians are sluggish to adopt treatment advances because of the perils of translating clinical trial recommendations

Rheum Dis Clin N Am 38 (2012) xi–xiv
http://dx.doi.org/10.1016/j.rdc.2012.10.001
0889-857X/12/$ – see front matter © 2012 Published by Elsevier Inc.

into clinical practice—exemplified by experiences with hormone replacement therapy, rofecoxib (Vioxx), rosiglitazone (Avandia), and thalidomide.[4]

Patients are also reluctant to change. When it comes to the utilization of novel therapies, Wolfe and Michaud have shown that patients prefer "the devil you know" (their current therapy) to "the devil you don't" (a new drug).[5] They found a sizeable discrepancy between the patient's treatment satisfaction and disease activity measures, which could be attributed to loss of disease control or fear of side effects.

If fear (or risk aversion) is the foundation of safety concerns, time, experience, and study may adjudicate safety concerns. Bringing a new drug to market in the United States may take 10 years and nearly a billion US dollars. Moreover, the conditions required for change may only evolve with long-term safety data. Hence, safety does not come cheaply, quickly, or easily. As a regulatory requirement for drug approval, pharmaceutical manufacturers are heavily invested in pharmacovigilance to ensure the long-term success of their product. Pharmacovigilance is the science of identifying, assessing, understanding, minimizing, and avoiding adverse effects and drug-related problems.[6] Global pharmacovigilance spending in 2010 was nearly $12 billion US. It begins during drug development (phase II and III trials) and is continued with long-term trials, postmarketing trials, widespread clinical use, medical reports of safety and efficacy, and population or registry-based observational studies. Indeed it is the frequent and pervasive focus on safety by many stakeholders that will establish the true safety and utility of a new agent.

The Food and Drug Administration (FDA) and other regulatory agencies are charged with ensuring the public health by ascertaining the safety, efficacy, and security of new medical interventions and products. These agencies have evolved to meet societal demands and commercial advancements as they impact population safety.[7] Recent changes at the FDA have focused on drug safety, especially with regard to product labeling clarity (boxed warnings, contraindications, warnings), postmarketing commitments by manufacturers (Risk Evaluation and Mitigation Strategies), and new initiatives designed to electronically gather more real-time information on drug safety at the time of approval (Sentinel Initiative).[8]

The safe use of drugs requires knowledge and experience but may also be bolstered by guidelines or rules. Chalkidou and coworkers[9] suggest that when considering new therapies we should ask the 3 following questions: (1) *Does current evidence suggest that the innovation is better than current practice?*; (2) *Is more information or study necessary?*; and (3) *Should we wait for more information?* Schiff and colleagues[2] have offered these principles for safe prescribing: (1) *think beyond drugs* (consider nondrug therapy; treatable underlying causes; and prevention); (2) *practice strategic prescribing* (defer nonurgent drug treatment; avoid unwarranted drug switching; be circumspect about unproven drug use; start treatment with only 1 new drug at a time; know who should not receive a drug); (3) *maintain heightened vigilance regarding adverse effects* (suspect drug reactions; be aware of withdrawal syndromes; and educate patients to anticipate reactions); (4) *exercise caution and skepticism regarding new drugs* (seek out unbiased information; wait until drugs have sufficient time on the market); (5) *work with patients for a shared agenda* (address nonadherence; patient preferences; education); and (6) *consider long-term, broader impacts* (weigh long-term outcomes and recognize that improved systems may outweigh marginal benefits of new drugs). Last, the clinician should recognize common pitfalls that include prescribing a drug: (1) *when no drug is needed*; (2) *when no drug is indicated*; (3) *that the drug is poorly chosen for the disease or patient*; (4) *that the drug is incorrectly dosed or used*; (5) *when no drug education or essential information is supplied*; (6) *when drugs are not monitored*; or (7) *when the patient is already receiving too many medications*.[10]

SUMMARY

This issue explores several important safety concerns that currently plague the rheumatologist and health care providers who care for patients with rheumatic diseases. Weighing safety against efficacy can be a complex task that is best alleviated by understanding the issues, nature, and breadth of problems associated with drug use. Therapeutic decision-making must be evidence-based, judicious, and appropriate for the patient and situation. Understanding drug safety is paramount to ensuring both success of therapy and benefit to the patient. Similarly, it is important not to underestimate the impact of uncontrolled disease activity in decision-making. Drug safety must be weighed against the severity and risks of the disease under treatment. Clearly the benefit/risk ratio has improved for many of the therapies discussed in this book.[11] The use of both conventional and novel therapies mandates an understanding of the mechanisms of action, unique toxicities, screening and monitoring measures, and rules for drug avoidance.

John J. Cush, MD
Baylor Research Institute
Baylor University Medical Center
Dallas, TX, USA

Kathryn H. Dao, MD
Baylor Research Institute
Dallas, TX, USA

E-mail addresses:
jjcush@gmail.com (J.J. Cush)
daokathryn@yahoo.com (K.H. Dao)

REFERENCES

1. Pisetsky D. Pisetsky's rules vs. the Peltzman effect: pondering drug safety. The Rheumatologist. 2009. Available at: http://www.the-rheumatologist.org/details/article/872139/Pisetskyrsquos_Rules_vs__the_Peltzman_Effect.html.
2. Schiff GD, Galanter WL, Duhig J, et al. Principles of conservative prescribing. Arch Intern Med 2011;171(16):1433–40.
3. Graham DJ, Ouellet-Hellstrom R, MaCurdy TE, et al. Risk of acute myocardial infarction, stroke, heart failure, and death in elderly Medicare patients treated with rosiglitazone or pioglitazone. JAMA 2010;304(4):411–8.
4. Lenfant C. Clinical research to clinical practice—lost in translation? N Engl J Med 2003;349:868–74.
5. Wolfe F, Michaud K. Resistance of rheumatoid arthritis patients to changing therapy: discordance between disease activity and patients' treatment choices. Arthritis Rheum 2007;56(7):2135–42.
6. The safety of medicines in public health programmes: pharmacovigilance: an essential tool. Geneva: WHO; 2006.
7. Hilts PJ. Protecting America's health: The FDA, business, and one hundred years of regulation. New York: Alfred A. Knopf; 2003.
8. Moore TJ, Singh S, Furberg CD. The FDA and new safety warnings. Arch Intern Med 2012;172(1):78–80.
9. Chalkidou K, Lord J, Fischer A, et al. Evidence-based decision making: when should we wait for more information? Health Aff 2008;27(6):1642–53.

10. Cush JJ, Kavanaugh A, Stein M. Prescribing guidelines. In: Cush JJ, Kavanaugh A, Stein M, editors. Rheumatology diagnosis and therapeutics. 2nd edition. Philadelphia: Lippincott Williams & Wilkins; 2005. p. 399–402.
11. Pincus T, Kavanaugh A, Sokka T. Benefit/risk of therapies for rheumatoid arthritis: underestimation of the "side effects" or risks of RA leads to underestimation of the benefit/risk of therapies. Clin Exp Rheumatol 2004;22(5 Suppl 35):S2–11.

Communicating the Risk of Side Effects to Rheumatic Patients

Richard W. Martin, MD, MA

KEYWORDS

- Risk communication • Decision support • Patient education • Quality of care
- Safety

KEY POINTS

- Every day in the clinic rheumatologists guide patients with decisions about initiating complex therapies.
- A good decision is informed, consistent with patient values and acted on.
- Cognitive biases, in part arising from reduced health literacy, can impair patient decision making.
- When sharing risk information, bias and framing effects can be in part accommodated by presenting absolute risks with supportive visual aids and context.
- Using decisions aids to structure and support deliberation after the office visit may improve patient decision making.

This monograph discusses the broad landscape of antirheumatic risks that rheumatologists must regularly address with patients. These include minor and serious adverse events, which may occur frequently or only rarely. Individual classes of medications (ie, disease-modifying antirheumatic drugs [DMARDs] or bisphosphonates) have unique risks and the target audience can vary greatly in demographics (ie, pregnancy, children–parental dyad, the elderly) or by circumstance (ie, at the time of surgery) in the setting of concurrent illnesses (ie, hepatitis C or latent tuberculosis). In some cases patient risk may vary based on individual characteristics and sometimes this tailored risk is known. In other cases only a global estimate of risk can be honestly offered. Despite incomplete data, for legal and ethical reasons, physicians must strive to inform patients about potential benefits and harms of medication options.

A good decision is informed, consistent with personal values, and acted on.[1] In an informed choice the decision maker understands relevant information and the choice reflects their values.[2] The capability of an individual patient to deliberate and their approaches to narrowing options and choosing may vary but an informed choice

Funding sources: None.
Conflict of interest: None.
Rheumatology, Department of Medicine, Michigan State University, College of Human Medicine, 1155 East Paris Northeast, Suite 100, Grand Rapids, MI 49546, USA
E-mail address: martin@mi-arthritis.com

should at least involve the patient in decision making to the extent they desire.[3] This can be assessed with the following questions[4]:

- Did the doctor make you aware of the different treatment options?
- Do you know the advantages and disadvantages of treatment or not having treatment?
- Are you adequately informed about the issues important to the decision?
- Has the doctor given you a chance to be involved in the decision?
- Do you believed an informed choice has been made?

There can be a gap between believing one is informed and actually being informed.[5,6] Being informed means knowing the options, being aware of the nature and frequency of the common and most serious medication risks and benefits. In addition, patients must know and be prepared to do the procedures for obtaining, administering, and keeping up with needed safety monitoring.

It is important to differentiate an informed choice from persuasion. Persuasion is a form of communication that is intentional; interpersonal; and involves creating, reinforcing, or modifying beliefs, intentions, motivations, or behaviors.[7] The overall goal is to influence the thoughts or actions of the decision maker.[8] In the case of many pharmaceutical advertisements, this may use symbolic expression, which emphasizes pictures instead of words. In addition, persuasive messages can appeal to fear (ie, of progression of rheumatoid arthritis [RA] joint damage) or protective motivation, which leads the patient to evaluate a health threat and their ability to cope and protect against the undesirable outcome. To illustrate these techniques, **Fig. 1** simulates a promotional message for a hypothetical DMARD. Typically, within industry promotional fliers (which are sometimes labeled "decision guides") there is a summary of risks displayed, but no estimates of the probability of outcomes or reference to other options. Specific information is printed on the "medication guide," which is tucked in a pocket in the back cover of the brochure.

In contrast, patient decision aids seek to support patients in making an informed choice by disclosing options and relevant information about the consequences of treatment in an accurate, balanced, and understandable manner. Patient decision aids then guide the consumer through steps to clarify the value they place on these

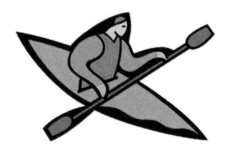

"If I knew then what I know now about Rheumatoid Arthritis, I would have been

more proactive."

Joan K - living with RA since 1990

Fig. 1. A hypothetical patient education brochure.

consequences.[9] This recognizes that in some decisions there is a need to portray equipoise.[10] This exists where there is a choice among two or more therapeutically equivalent options. Based on medical evidence, the professional may have no preferred recommendation; however, individual treatment attributes or outcomes may be more important or valued by an individual patient. Consider the choice of a bisphosphonate for osteoporosis. Patients must make a trade-off between cost, convenience, hassle of administration, and gastrotoxicity when choosing among a generic oral, once weekly, a branded oral, once monthly, and a branded, intravenous, yearly agent. The expected increase in bone density and fracture risk may be the same; however, inconveniences, costs, and risk of toxicity do vary among the choices. Thus, when equipoise exists, the deciding factors should be the patient's personal values and preferences related to the potential outcomes of treatment. However, to be aware of one's preferences, a patient must be informed of treatment options and outcomes, have the time and ability to reflect, and in some cases need structured support to clarify what they believe are the factors that are to them most important.

As patients consider options and choose they may use one or more cognitive strategies. Prospect theory suggests that decision makers carefully weigh multiple attributes of available treatment options before arriving at a rational choice that maximizes benefit.[11] Kahneman,[12] a Nobel laureate in economics, describes that as relying on "System 2," which is the mode of thinking that directs conscious, deliberate, effortful activities, such as choice. Alternatively, patients may use a heuristic approach, making simpler more cognitively efficient decisions using rules of thumb. Kahneman labels this as directed by "System 1," which is the mode of thinking that is unconscious, fast, intuitive, and the source of impressions and feelings at the source of many explicit beliefs.[12] Many decisions made by patients and expert physicians are heuristic based. However, the way in which people process information and use personal heuristics can introduce cognitive bias in decision making and lead to suboptimal decisions.[13]

Patient characteristics can also influence decision making. Age and general health can effect concentration and cognition, which are necessary in making good decisions.[14,15] Health literacy is a measure of multiple domains, including reading; ability to locate and use information; and doing simple mathematical tasks (numeracy). Health literacy is influenced not only by formal education but also by cognitive function including recall and critical thinking.[16] In a survey of a large cohort of community patients with RA it was found that health literacy, independent of low educational achievement or other demographic, was a common predictor of risk perception and willingness to take a proposed DMARD.[17] In addition, it was observed that risk perception was increased by negative RA disease and treatment experience, whereas willingness to take a proposed DMARD was reduced as perception of current RA control improved. This demonstrates the influences of patient disease experiences on decision-making processes. These findings are consistent with the observations of other investigators that individuals with low numeracy may have a higher susceptibility to information-framing effects.[18] In addition, they may be less effective or exert less effort trying to decode medication information and more likely to rely on established heuristics; rules of thumb, such as "if I had a side effect before, it will happen again"; or antidotal reasoning.[13]

Mood is another potentially important patient characteristic. There is evidence that a depressed person's diminished ability to think and concentrate or indecisiveness may impair ability to participate in decision making.[19] However, in a study of community patients with RA, no significant effect of depression or happiness on risk perception or willingness to take a proposed DMARD was found.[17] This confirms previous observations in a separate RA cohort that history of major depression was not significantly related to patient satisfaction with decision.[20]

Finally, an understudied area is the effect of the doctor-patient interaction on treatment decisions. In a previous study it was found that patients' trust in their rheumatologist had nearly seven times the effect on their confidence in a DMARD decision than any other predictor including numeric literacy and DMARD-related knowledge.[21] This supports the position that despite physicians' efforts to educate, many patients make decisions based on factors that are peripheral to the substance of health information and focus on clues, such as physician characteristics of goodwill, expertise, or trustworthiness, when choosing a medication.

If a good decision is dependent on an individual's ability to understand and evaluate options and to make judgments that are relatively free of bias,[22] then physicians should consider if individual patient characteristics may complicate comprehension. Physicians often overestimate patient literacy[23] and because of unawareness or shame if not questioned, patients may not disclose their limitation.[24] This may justify routine health literacy screening to identify patients who need low literacy materials or consider using enhanced strategies to support patient decision making. Fortunately, there are simple methods, such as screening questions and word recognition tests, that make routine screening for low or marginal health literacy feasible in the clinic.[25,26]

As physicians consider how to present information about risks of treatment, several general and specific considerations arise. In general, the context and framing of a decision can be important. For example, in the presentation of economic risk, the endowment effect has been observed where individuals are motivated by the possibility of losing more than gaining something of value. This "I would have been" framing is the persuasive approach in the industry medication message cited previously. It is also known as a negativity bias or loss aversion. Interestingly, meta-analysis evaluating such framing studies in health messages has unexpectedly failed to show a persuasive advantage for this loss-frame approach in health-related messages.[27] Thus, cognitive bias may in some cases be domain specific. Another example of potentially motivating and biasing communication is using personal stories or testimonials that illustrate other patients' interpretation of decision experiences. Most rheumatologists recall persuasive advertisements with testimonials recommending the use of etanercept by public figures, such as golfer Phil Nicholson or the grandson of the famous aviator Charles Lindberg. In general, personal stories that emphasize specific reasons for a choice or introduce emotional terms may introduce bias, whereas stories that illustrate how others made sense about the facts may aid informed decision making.[28] A good use of patient narratives is illustrated in the design of the UK National Health Service direct decision aid for patients considering treatments of osteoarthritis of the knee (https://www.nhsdirect.nhs.uk/DecisionAids/PDAs/PDA_KneeArthritis.aspx).

Physicians should provide patients with information about treatment options and the possible benefits and side effects. For several years the rheumatology faculty at Michigan State University has used decision aids developed to support the discussion of antirheumatics and structure patient deliberation after the office visit.[29–31] Although these types of decision supports may not be necessary in all medication discussions, readers may wish to review them (www.mi-arthritis.com) as specific exemplars that meet the International Patient Decision Aids Standards for high-quality decision aids.[32] They begin by directly stating the decision to be made. Background about RA, available treatments, and the expected course of RA with or without treatment are outlined. Next presented is specific information regarding the medication recommended by the rheumatologist. This includes the most common or serious side effects. Described are individual medication side effects and what it would be like to experience them. For example, a serious infection is described in this way[29]: "Because MTX reduces the hyperactive immune system in RA, it can also reduce your ability to fight off serious infections like pneumonia, kidney infections, etc. When we refer to serious infections, we mean infections severe enough that you would need to be admitted to the hospital for one or more days to receive antibiotics through the vein and/or other care like IV fluids and oxygen." It is essential for a patient to comprehend the personal impact of a side effect to be able to construct a meaningful value to that possible outcome.

Next presented is the probability of important outcomes. Several basic principles have been recognized as best practices in communicating risk.[5,33] The first is to present frequency of a risk as an absolute risk rather than relative risk.[34] Presenting relative risk tends to inflate the perceived benefits of therapy.[35] For example, a hypothetical drug may reduce the relative risk of fracture by 40%. However, if this represents an absolute risk reduction from 1% per year to 0.6% per year a patient may interpret this as a lesser benefit. Another approach is to offer patients information as natural frequencies rather than probabilities,[36] which in essence "does the math" by deconstructing the probability. Visual aids, such as natural frequency trees (**Fig. 2**) or pictographs, may reduce some bias and framing effects and aid the understanding of incremental risk (**Fig. 3**). One should also attempt to communicate the uncertainty around numeric risks presented. The estimates presented in decision aids from the University of Ottawa describe the source and quality of risk estimates as very low (+) to high (++++). Other designers qualify risk statements as "roughly 2 in 100". Han and coworkers[37] take the sophisticated approach of presenting a random pictogram, which can be animated (**Fig. 4**). In some cases it is possible to present more patient-specific or tailored outcome information. Another approach demonstrated in the University of Ottawa "stepped decision aid" addresses a need to give information tailored to the stage of disease (http://decisionaid.ohri.ca/decaids.html). The patient answers questions about their impairment from osteoarthritis, and from this they are classified into level 0 to 5 disease. Patients then can review treatment options relevant for their level of disease, and the specific benefits and harms for each. **Box 1** illustrates another tailored approach used by Dr David Hickman of Oregon Health Sciences University in an Agency for Healthcare Research and Quality funded decision aid that presented age-specific risk of gastrointestinal bleeding. In some cases one must communicate rate of outcome rather than frequency of outcome. For example, if RA or systemic lupus erythematosis is not treated, continuing disease activity may lead to progression of end organ damage. When communicating rate of disease progression it may be preferred to use speedometers rather than a pictograph.[31] **Fig. 5** is an excerpt from a methotrexate decision aid that describes how RA joint damage is slowed with treatment.[29] To ensure patients understand the link between clinical arthritis and the progression of joint damage both are contrasted over time. In addition, the effect of methotrexate in percent absolute

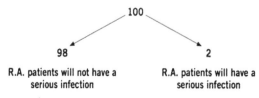

Fig. 2. Natural frequency tree.

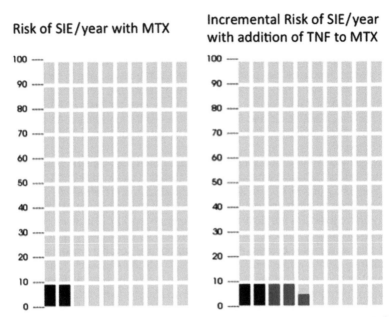

Fig. 3. Simple and incremental risk pictograms. MTX, methotrexate; SIE, serious infectious event; TNF, tumor necrosis factor.

reduction of rate of progression followed by speedometers that contrast the progression of joint damage without and with methotrexate therapy are described.

Finally, if patients use rational decision-making processes they consider the likelihood of treatment outcomes, including potential benefits and harms, and how important these outcomes are to them. Economists and policy makers determine societal-based values or utilities of outcomes and integrate this information using decision analysis[38–40] or Markov models[41] to identify dominant treatment strategies.

Communicating Randomness of Risk

Non-random pictograph

Lifetime Risk: 9.0%
Explanation: Based on the information provided, the estimated chance for developing colorectal cancer over the lifetime is 9%.

We can't predict the future of any one person. Risk estimates only tell us **how many** people in a population are likely to get colon cancer; they can't tell us **who** will get the disease or not.

Random, static pictograph

Lifetime Risk: 9.0%
Explanation: Based on the information provided, the estimated chance for developing colorectal cancer over the lifetime is 9%.

We can't predict the future of any one person. Risk estimates only tell us **how many** people in a population are likely to get colon cancer; they can't tell us **who** will get the disease or not.

Fig. 4. Communicating randomness of risk. (*Adapted from* Han PK, Klein W, Killam B, et al. Representing randomness in the communication of individualized cancer risk estimates: effects on cancer risk perceptions, worry, and subjective uncertainty about risk. Patient Educ Couns 2012;86:106–13; with permission.)

Box 1
Tailored risk of gastrointestinal bleeding from nonsteroidal anti-inflammatories drugs (NSAIDs)

In general, stomach bleeding is more likely for people taking NSAIDs who:

- Are older, especially more than 75 years old
- Take higher doses
- Use NSAIDs for a longer time.
- Also take medicine to help prevent blood clots, like aspirin or warfarin (Coumadin®).
- Older people taking NSAID pills have higher risk of stomach bleeding
- For people age 16–44:
  - 5 out of 10,000 people taking NSAIDs will have a serious bleed
  - 1 out of 10,000 people taking NSAIDs will die from a bleed
- For people age 45–64:
  - 15 out of 10,000 people taking NSAIDs will have a serious bleed
  - 2 out of 10,000 people taking NSAIDs will die from a bleed
- For people age 65–74:
  - 17 out of 10,000 people taking NSAIDs will have a serious bleed
  - 3 out of 10,000 people taking NSAIDs will die from a bleed
- For people age 75 or older:
  - 91 out of 10,000 people taking NSAIDs will have a serious bleed
  - 15 out of 10,000 people taking NSAIDs will die from a bleed

Data from AHRQ. Clinician guide: choosing non-opioid analgesics for osteoarthritis. AHRQ Publication Number 06(07)-EHC009-2A.

However, when supporting an individual patient making a decision, the physician is more concerned with helping that patient clarify what outcomes matter to them the most. Preferences[42] and outcome importance ranking might be directly elicited with visual analogue scales, as is the approach in the Ottawa Generic Personal Decision Guide (**Fig. 6**).[43] Alternatively, more complex computer-based survey methods have been used, such as analytic hierarchy process[44] and conjoint analysis.[45] For clinicians, simply engaging the patient with a question, such as "are there any side effects

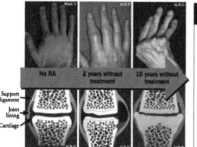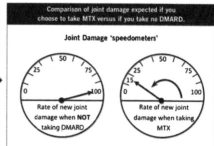

Fig. 5. Communicating rate of disease progression. (*Data from* Martin RW, Gallager PJ, Eggebeen AT, et al. A decision aid for rheumatoid arthritis patients considering methotrexate therapy. Arthritis Rheum 2009;60:S324.)

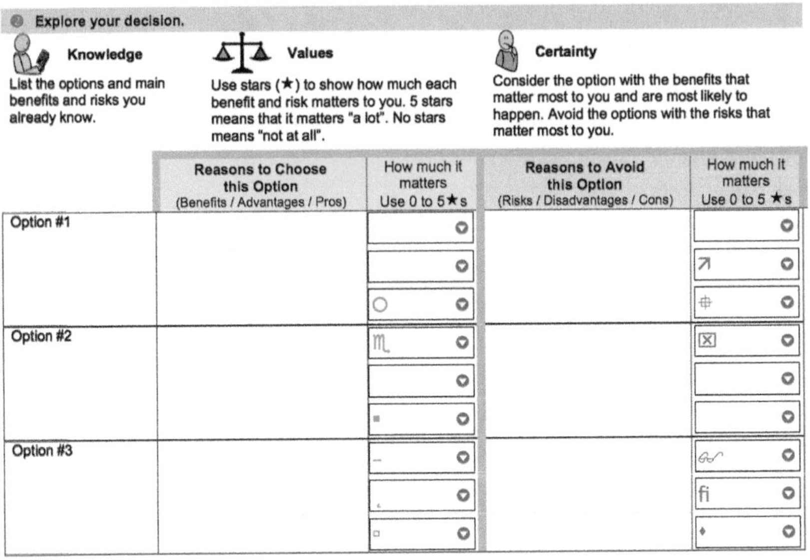
Explore your decision.

Knowledge
List the options and main benefits and risks you already know.

Values
Use stars (★) to show how much each benefit and risk matters to you. 5 stars means that it matters "a lot". No stars means "not at all".

Certainty
Consider the option with the benefits that matter most to you and are most likely to happen. Avoid the options with the risks that matter most to you.

	Reasons to Choose this Option (Benefits / Advantages / Pros)	How much it matters Use 0 to 5★s	Reasons to Avoid this Option (Risks / Disadvantages / Cons)	How much it matters Use 0 to 5 ★s
Option #1				
Option #2				
Option #3				

Fig. 6. Preference elicitation: Ottawa generic personal decision guide. (Ottawa Personal Decision Guide © 2012 O'Connor, Stacey, Jacobsen. Ottawa Hospital Research Institute and University of Ottawa, Canada.)

that particularly concern you," may lead to a conversation that helps the patient become aware of what matters to them the most. Whatever elicitation technique used, if the patient has had satisfactory review of accurate, balanced information regarding the risks and benefits of reasonable treatment options, and then makes a choice that matches their personal values, then the physician has succeeded in facilitating a good decision.

REFERENCES

1. O'Connor AM. Ottawa decision support framework. Ottawa (Canada): Cochrane Musculoskeletal Review Group; 2006.
2. Marteau T. Informed choice: a construct in search of a name. In: Edwards A, Elywn G, editors. Shared decision-making in health care. 2nd edition. Oxford (United Kingdom): Oxford University Press; 2009. p. 87–93.
3. Edwards A, Elwyn G. Inside the black box of shared decision making: distinguishing between the process of involvement and who makes the decision. Health Expect 2006;9(4):307–20.
4. Edwards A, Elwyn G, Hood K, et al. The development of COMRADE–a patient-based outcome measure to evaluate the effectiveness of risk communication and treatment decision making in consultations. Patient Educ Couns 2003;50(3):311–22.
5. Feldman-Stewart D, O'Brien MA, Clayman M, et al. Providing information about options. International Patient Decision Aid Standards Collaboration Background Document; 2012.
6. Sepucha KR, Fagerlin A, Couper MP, et al. How does feeling informed relate to being informed? The DECISIONS survey. Med Decis Making 2010;30(Suppl 5):77S–84S.

7. Gass RH, Seiter JS. Persuasion, social influence, and compliance gaining. 3rd edition. Boston: Pearson; 2007.

8. Cameron KA. A practitioner's guide to persuasion: an overview of 15 selected persuasion theories, models and frameworks. Patient Educ Couns 2009;74(3): 309–17.

9. O'Connor AM, Edwards A. The role of decision aids in promoting evidence-based patient choice. In: Edwards AE, Elwynn, G, editors. Shared decision-making in health care. 2nd edition. Oxford (United Kingdom): Oxford University Press; 2009. p. 191–200.

10. Elwyn G, Edwards A, Kinnersley P, et al. Shared decision making and the concept of equipoise: the competences of involving patients in healthcare choices. Br J Gen Pract 2000;50(460):892–9.

11. Kahneman D, Tversky A. Prospect theory: an analysis decision under risk. In: Kahneman D, Tversky A, editors. Choices, values and frames. Cambridge (United Kingdom): Cambridge University Press; 2000. p. 17–43.

12. Kahneman D. Thinking, fast and slow. New York: Farrar, Straus and Giroux; 2011.

13. Fagerlin A, Wang C, Ubel PA. Reducing the influence of anecdotal reasoning on people's health care decisions: is a picture worth a thousand statistics? Med Decis Making 2005;25(4):398–405.

14. Shin SY, Katz P, Wallhagen M, et al. Cognitive impairment in persons with rheumatoid arthritis. Arthritis Care Res (Hoboken) 2012;64:1144–50.

15. Finucane ML, Slovic P, Hibbard JH, et al. Aging and decision-making competence: an analysis of comprehension and consistency skills in older versus younger adults considering health-plan options. J Behav Decis Making 2002; 15:141–64.

16. Jensen J. Addressing health literacy in the design of health messages. In: Cho H, editor. Health communication message design. Thousand Oaks (CA): Sage; 2012. p. 171–4.

17. Martin RW, Head AJ, Eggebeen AT, et al. Does Biased Risk Perception Explain the Underuse of Disease Modifying Anti-Rheumatic Drugs? Arthritis Rheum 2012;64:S627.

18. Peters E. Beyond comprehension: the role of numeracy in judgements and decisions. Curr Dir Psychol Sci 2012;21:31–5.

19. Loh A, Leonhart R, Wills CE, et al. The impact of patient participation on adherence and clinical outcome in primary care of depression. Patient Educ Couns 2007;65(1):69–78.

20. Martin RW, Holmes-Rovner MK, Raykov T. Does depression modify patient appraisal of anti-rheumatic drug treatment effects? Pittsburgh: Society for Medical Decision Making; 2007.

21. Martin RW, Head AJ, Rene J, et al. Patient decision-making related to antirheumatic drugs in rheumatoid arthritis: the importance of patient trust of physician. J Rheumatol 2008;35(4):618–24.

22. Leykin Y, Roberts CS, Derubeis RJ. Decision-making and depressive symptomatology. Cognit Ther Res 2011;35(4):333–41.

23. Kelly PA, Haidet P. Physician overestimation of patient literacy: a potential source of health care disparities. Patient Educ Couns 2007;66:119–22.

24. Parikh NS, Parker RM, Nurss JR, et al. Shame and health literacy: the unspoken connection. Patient Educ Couns 1996;27:33–9.

25. Chew LD, Griffin JM, Partin MR, et al. Validation of screening questions for limited health literacy in a large VA outpatient population. J Gen Intern Med 2008;23(5): 561–6.

26. Martin RW, Bater R, Head AJ, et al. Identifying patients who need low literacy materials to support anti-rheumatic drug decision making. Arthritis Rheum 2007;56:S109.

27. O'Keefe D. From psychology theory to message design. In: Cho H, editor. Health communication message design. Thousand Oaks (CA): Sage; 2012. p. 3–20.

28. Bekker HL, Winterbottom A, Foweler V, et al. Using personal stories. 2012 Update of the International Patient Decision Aid Standards Collaboration Background Document. 2012.

29. Martin RW, Gallager PJ, Eggebeen AT, et al. A decision aid for rheumatoid arthritis patients considering methotrexate therapy. Arthritis Rheum 2009;60:S324.

30. Martin RW, Lajevardi N, Sevak S, et al. Placing serious infection risk in perspective. A randomized trial evaluating a patient decision aid to reduce focusing illusion. Arthritis Rheum 2011;63:S275.

31. Martin RW, Brower ME, Geralds A, et al. An experimental evaluation of patient decision aid design to communicate the effects of medications on the rate of progression of structural joint damage in rheumatoid arthritis. Patient Educ Couns 2012;86(3):329–34.

32. Elwyn G, O'Connor A, Stacey D, et al. Developing a quality criteria framework for patient decision aids: online international Delphi consensus process. BMJ 2006; 333(7565):417.

33. Fagerlin A, Zikmund-Fisher BJ, Ubel PA. Helping patients decide: ten steps to better risk communication. J Natl Cancer Inst 2011;103(19):1436–43.

34. Schwartz LM, Woloshin S, Welch HG. The drug facts box: providing consumers with simple tabular data on drug benefit and harm. Med Decis Making 2007; 27(5):655–62.

35. Schwartz LM, Woloshin S, Welch HG. Using a drug facts box to communicate drug benefits and harms: two randomized trials. Ann Intern Med 2009;150(8): 516–27.

36. Trevena L, Zikmund-Fisher B, Edwards A, et al. Presenting probabilities about options. International Patient Decision Aid Standards Collaboration Background Document: International Patient Decision Aid Standards Collaboration. 2012.

37. Han PK, Klein W, Killam B, et al. Representing randomness in the communication of individualized cancer risk estimates: effects on cancer risk perceptions, worry, and subjective uncertainty about risk. Patient Educ Couns 2012;86:106–13.

38. Detsky AS, Naglie G, Krahn MD, et al. Primer on medical decision analysis. Part 1: getting started. Med Decis Making 1997;17(2):123–5.

39. Detsky AS, Naglie G, Krahn MD, et al. Primer on medical decision analysis. Part 2: building a tree. Med Decis Making 1997;17(2):126–35.

40. Krahn MD, Naglie G, Naimark D, et al. Primer on medical decision analysis. Part 4: analyzing the model and interpreting the results. Med Decis Making 1997;17(2):142–51.

41. Naimark D, Krahn MD, Naglie G, et al. Primer on medical decision analysis. Part 5: working with Markov processes. Med Decis Making 1997;17(2):152–9.

42. Naglie G, Krahn MD, Naimark D, et al. Primer on medical decision analysis. Part 3: estimating probabilities and utilities. Med Decis Making 1997;17(2):136–41.

43. O'Connor AM, Stacey D, Jacobsen MJ. Ottawa personal decision guide. Ottawa (Canada): Ottawa Hospital Research Institute & University of Ottawa; 2012.

44. Dolan JG. Shared decision-making–transferring research into practice: the Analytic Hierarchy Process. Patient Educ Couns 2008;73(3):418–25.

45. Fraenkel L. Conjoint analysis at the individual patient level: issues to consider as we move from a research to a clinical tool. Patient 2008;1(4):251–3.

Safety of Urate-Lowering Therapies
Managing the Risks to Gain the Benefits

Robert T. Keenan, MD, MPH[a,b,*]

KEYWORDS

- Gout • Allopurinol • Febuxostat • Pelgoticase • Safety

KEY POINTS

- Safe use of urate-lowering therapy in patients with gout with multiple comorbidities can be a challenge for the clinician.
- Potential drug-drug interactions between traditional urate-lowering therapies and frequently prescribed medications are more common than usually appreciated, but can be appropriately managed in most patients.
- Allopurinol and other urate-lowering therapies can be safely used in patients with renal disease and other comorbidities.
- New therapies have provided additional options for patients with gout that may allow for safer and better management of their disease.

INTRODUCTION

Gout is the most common inflammatory arthropathy affecting more than 8 million adults in the United States alone.[1] The prevalence of gout continues to increase in the United States as well as abroad.[2,3] Gout affects more than 6 million men and more than 2 million women, and the rising incidence parallels with conditions such as cardiovascular (CV) disease, metabolic syndrome, chronic kidney disease (CKD), and an aging population.[4–6] This association is unlikely coincidental, as there is accumulating evidence suggestive of gout potentially contributing to a number of the aforementioned comorbidities.[7,8] Regardless of whether or not gout plays a causative role, the fact patients with gout frequently have multiple comorbidities is undisputable.[9–12]

Financial disclosure: Consultant: Savient Pharmaceuticals; Speakers Bureau: Savient Pharmaceuticals; Research Support: Novartis Pharmaceuticals.
[a] Duke Gout and Crystal Arthropathies Clinic, Duke Specialty Infusion Center, 50 Medicine Drive, Durham, NC 27710, USA; [b] Division of Rheumatology and Immunology, Department of Medicine, Duke University School of Medicine, Durham, NC 27710, USA
* Duke University Medical Center, 200 Trent Drive, DUMC 3544, Durham, NC.
E-mail address: robert.keenan@duke.edu

Rheum Dis Clin N Am 38 (2012) 663–680
http://dx.doi.org/10.1016/j.rdc.2012.08.008
0889-857X/12/$ – see front matter © 2012 Elsevier Inc. All rights reserved.

With the increase in the incidence and prevalence of gout, new urate-lowering therapies (ULT) have become available and a renaissance of interest in gout has occurred. Forty years after the introduction of allopurinol (Aloprim; Zyloprim) and 50 years after probenecid (Benemid),[13,14] febuxostat (Uloric) and pegloticase (Krystexxa) have been added to the arsenal against gout. Yet despite the surge in gout interest and new therapies, there is substantial evidence that quality of gout care continues to be inadequate. Patients with gout have been repeatedly shown to have greater morbidity compared with their counterparts without gout.[9,15–18] In some patients, hyperuricemia and gout may be simply a prelude for impending illnesses; but often, by the time a patient is diagnosed with gout, comorbidities are well established and are being treated with multiple medications.

Managing gout is intrinsically straightforward. The goal is to reduce and maintain serum urate (SU) levels well below that of physiologic supersaturation (6.8 mg/dL). Maintaining SU levels below this level allows for the mobilization of monosodium urate crystals out of joints and soft tissue, eventually eliminating the nidus of acute and chronic inflammation. As lower SU levels directly correlate with an increased rate by which tophi resolve,[19] using a target goal of less than 6 mg/dL as a starting point can decrease and ideally eliminate the crystal burden, thereby eradicating tophi and future flares. With appropriate therapy and compliance, most patients with gout should be able to achieve full remission. Challenges arise when clinicians and patients are faced with potential adverse drug reactions (ADRs) owing to decreased renal clearance, hepatic impairment, drug-drug interactions, or simply, intolerance.[9]

All Food and Drug Administration (FDA)-approved medications have risks and benefits. It is paramount to consider potential pitfalls and benedictions of a therapy before its use. Both the provider and the patient must balance a medication's risks and benefits to determine if it is the safest and most efficacious option. It is also important to understand the risk of any therapy for an individual patient is not static; rather it is a dynamic process that involves pharmacokinetics, pharmacodynamics (PD), and drug-drug interactions.[20] This article reviews the safety of current ULT indicated for the use of chronic gout, including allopurinol, febuxostat, pegloticase, and probenecid. Monitoring practices and strategies to decrease the risk of potential adverse effects in clinical practice are also reviewed.

BURDEN OF GOUT AND ADVERSE DRUG REACTIONS

The cost of ADRs caused by all medications is estimated to account for 5% to 9% of all inpatient costs.[21] There is little data regarding the impact of gout therapy–specific ADRs on patient disability and health care costs. Conversely, it has been shown that inadequately treated patients with gout have a poorer quality of life versus their age-matched and comorbidity-matched peers. Also, the annual direct and indirect costs of having gout are estimated to range from $800 to $10,000.[22–24] The impact of gout on the quality of life and potential economic burden emphasizes the importance of treating these patients appropriately and safely.

XANTHINE OXIDASE INHIBITORS
Allopurinol

There has been a renewed surge in the medical management of chronic gout with the development of several new therapies. Even in this light, allopurinol has seemed to have a rebirth of its own. Initially developed as an antineoplastic agent in the mid-1950s, allopurinol is a purine analog, an isomer of hypoxanthine, which inhibits xanthine oxidase. Allopurinol is the most commonly prescribed ULT, and continues to be the foundation and benchmark for chronic gout therapy since its approval by the FDA in 1966.[13,25] The half-life of allopurinol in the blood is short (1.1 ± 0.3 hour), and is rapidly metabolized to its active metabolite, oxypurinol. In contrast to allopurinol, oxypurinol has a relatively long half-life (23 ± 7 hours), and is largely responsible for urate reduction.[26] Given its long half-life and noncompetitive inhibition of xanthine oxidase, oxypurinol has been deemed the perpetrator of intolerance and ADRs associated with allopurinol use.

Drug-drug interactions
Both allopurinol and oxypurinol inhibit xanthine oxidase, therefore concomitant use of medications such as azathioprine and mercaptopurine, which are also metabolized by xanthine oxidase or inhibit xanthine oxidase, should be used with caution. There are several known allopurinol-drug interactions of which the clinician should be aware when making therapeutic decisions (**Table 1**). There have been case reports suggesting interactions between allopurinol and some classes of antihypertensive medications, including angiotensin-converting enzyme inhibitors and diuretics (see later in this article), but a causal relationship has not been proven.[27–29]

Adverse drug reactions
Allopurinol is generally well tolerated, but up to 5% of patients stop the medication because of any ADR.[30] Common side effects include gout flares, nausea, diarrhea, pruritis, and approximately 2% of patients develop a mild rash. Less commonly, allopurinol can cause vomiting, hepatitis, agranulocytosis, and headache. When starting any ULT, the risk of flares should be discussed with the patient, and appropriate prophylaxis should be started 1 to 2 weeks before initiating therapy (eg, colchicine, nonsteroidal anti-inflammatories [NSAIDs]) (**Table 2**).

The side-effect profile is no worse than most medications prescribed on a regular basis by clinicians, but there is still reluctance to use allopurinol, especially at dosages appropriate to decrease SU levels below the limit of solubility (and therefore prevent further formation and facilitate dissolution of tophi). The basis of this reluctancy is because of a rare, but potentially fatal, ADR known as allopurinol hypersensitivity syndrome (AHS). The estimated incidence of AHS is 0.1% to 0.4%, and the mortality rate is 5% to 30%, depending on the severity. This rare, but potentially lethal, syndrome is characterized by a constellation of signs and symptoms (**Box 1**).[31,32]

Risk factors for AHS include female sex, age, genetic disposition, recent commencement of allopurinol, diuretic use, and renal impairment.[33,34] ADRs and AHS usually occur within days to weeks after initiation of allopurinol, with a median of approximately 30 days and 90% occurring within 180 days.[30,35] As more men are prescribed allopurinol, most AHS cases have been male, but multiple analyses have shown women may be more at risk than men.[30,31,35] Age may also increase the risk of AHA, especially mortality associated with AHA. This is thought to be because of several factors, including decreased renal clearance, increased diuretic use, and comorbidities.[35,36]

There is a growing body of evidence that genetics plays a significant role in severe drug reactions. The role of the major histocompatibility complex type I allele, HLA-B*5801, has been shown in several studies to increase the risk for AHS.[33,37–40] In a case-control analysis of Han Chinese, 100% of patients with AHS carried the allele versus 15% of patients who tolerated the medication, resulting in an odds ratio of 580 (95% confidence interval, 34–9780).[37] Hung and colleagues suggested that the HLA-B*5801 allele was necessary, but not sufficient for AHS to occur. Similarly, in a recent analysis in a Thai population, 100% of patients with AHS carried HLA-B*5801, whereas only 13% of the control patients carried it, yielding an odds ratio of 348 (95% confidence interval, 19–6336).[37]

Table 1
ULT-drug interactions

Drug	Risk Rating	Risk	Reliability Rating
Allopurinol-Drug Interaction			
ACE inhibitors	D	Possible increased risk of allergy/hypersensitivity	Fair
Amoxicillin/ampicillin	C	Possible increased risk of allergy/hypersensitivity	Fair
Antacids[a]	D	Decrease absorption of allopurinol	Good
Azathioprine	D	Accumulation of mercaptopurine/increased risk of toxicity/bone marrow suppression	Fair
Mercaptopurine	D	Accumulation of mercaptopurine/increased risk of toxicity/bone marrow suppression	Fair
Phenytoin	C	Increased serum levels of phenytoin	Fair
Carbamazepine	C	Increased serum levels of carbamazepine	Fair
Cyclophosphamide	C	Increased cyclophosphamide levels/Increased risk of bone marrow suppression	Good
Cyclosporine	D	Increased cyclosporine levels/Increased risk of bone marrow suppression	Poor
Didanosine	X	Increased didanosine levels and toxicity	Good
Loop diuretics	C	Possible increased risk of allergy/hypersensitivity[b]	Fair
Thiazide diuretics	C	Possible increased risk of allergy/hypersensitivity[b]	Fair
Theophylline derivatives	C	Increased levels of theophylline	Good
Warfarin	D	May enhance anticoagulant effect of warfarin and other vitamin K antagonists	Good
Febuxostat-Drug Interaction			
Azathioprine	X	Accumulation of mercaptopurine/increased risk of toxicity/bone marrow suppression	Fair
Mercaptopurine	X	Accumulation of mercaptopurine/increased risk of toxicity/bone marrow suppression	Fair
Didanosine	X	Increased didanosine levels and toxicity	Fair

Theophylline derivatives	C	Increased levels of theophylline metabolite	Fair
Pegloticase-Drug Interaction			
Pegylated drug products	C	Possibly diminish clinical response to pegylated drug if used together	Poor
Other urate-lowering therapy	X	May lower serum urate level in patient NOT responding to pegloticase, which increases the risk for infusion reaction or anaphylaxis	Fair
Probenecid-Drug Interaction			
Methotrexate	D	May increase serum concentration of methotrexate	Excellent
Mycophenolate mofetil	D	May increase levels of mycophenolate and increase risk of toxicity	Fair
Nonsteroidal anti-inflammatory agents	C	May increase the serum concentration of nonsteroidals	Good
Salicylates	C	May diminish therapeutic effect of probenecid	Excellent
Penicillin	C	May increase effects of penicillins; consider avoiding use in renal insufficiency	Excellent
Zidovudine	C	May decrease metabolism of zidovudine and increase risk for toxicity	Excellent

Risk Rating[74]: C, Monitor Therapy: The benefits of concomitant use of these 2 medications usually outweigh the risks. An appropriate monitoring plan should be implemented to identify potential negative effects. Dosage adjustments of 1 or both agents may be needed in a minority of patients.

D, Consider Therapy Modification: Patient-specific assessment must be conducted to determine whether the benefits of concomitant therapy outweigh the risks. Specific actions must be taken to realize the benefits and/or minimize the toxicity resulting from concomitant use. Aggressive monitoring, empiric dosage changes, choosing alternative agents, may be indicated.

X, Avoid Combination: The risks associated with concomitant use of these agents usually outweigh the benefits. These agents are generally considered contra-indicated with concomitant use.

Reliability Rating[74]: Poor, <2 case reports with no other supporting data or theoretical. Fair, >2 case reports; or <2 case reports with other supporting data. Good, single randomized, controlled clinical trial (RCT). Excellent, multiple RCTs; or single RCT plus >2 case reports.

Abbreviation: ACE, angiotensin-converting enzyme.

[a] Except sodium bicarbonate.

[b] See text.

Adapted from Refs.[61,71,74,75]

Table 2
Urate-lowering therapy cautions, contraindications, and prevention

	Indication	Caution	Risk Prevention	Contraindication
Allopurinol	Management of hyperuricemia in patients with gout	Acute gout flare; Renal insufficiency[a]; Hepatic impairment	Prophylactic therapy (eg, colchicine), initiate 1–2 wk prior; Start at low dose and titrate up; monitor CBC, hepatic function every 4–8 wk	Hypersensitivity; Concomitant use with azathioprine, mercaptopurine
Febuxostat	Management of hyperuricemia in patients with gout	Acute gout flare; History of CVD[a], Hepatic impairment	Prophylactic therapy (eg, colchicine), initiate 1–2 wk prior; Start at low dose; monitor CBC, hepatic function every 8–12 wk	Hypersensitivity; Concomitant use with azathioprine, mercaptopurine
Pegloticase	Refractory chronic gout	Acute gout flare; Heart failure[a]; Infusion reaction; Owing to premedication with corticosteroids, caution should be used in diabetes mellitus, heart failure[a]	Prophylactic therapy (eg, colchicine), initiate 1–2 wk prior; ensure heart failure is compensated; monitor SU levels <24–48 h before second and subsequent infusions; [monitor and/or have patients adjust diabetes medications as needed]	G6PD deficiency; Uncompensated heart failure (uncontrolled CVD); 1 or 2 consecutive SU levels >6 mg/dL; Hypersensitivity reaction[a], concomitant use of other ULT
Probenecid	Management of hyperuricemia in patients with gout	Acute gout flares; renal insufficiency; history of urate stones; G6PD deficiency	Prophylactic therapy (eg, colchicine), initiate 1–2 wk prior; Start low dose and titrate up slowly; monitor CBC, renal function every 4–6 wk	Hypersensitivity; blood dyscrasias, chronic urate stones

Abbreviations: CBC, complete blood count; CVD, cardiovascular disease; G6PD, glucose-6-phosphate dehydrogenase deficiency; SU, serum urate; ULT, urate-lowering therapy.

[a] See text.

Box 1
Allopurinol hypersensitivity syndrome: criteria and clinical manifestations

1. Clear history of exposure to allopurinol

2. Clinical presentation including

    a. At least 2 of the following major criteria

        i. Renal failure

        ii. Acute hepatocellular injury

        iii. Severe rash (Stevens Johnson syndrome, toxic epidermal necrolysis, or a diffuse exanthematous or exfoliative dermatitis

    Or

    b. 1 of the major criteria plus at least 1 of the following minor criteria:

        i. Fever

        ii. Eosinophilia

        iii. Leukocytosis

3. No history of exposure to another drug that may cause a similar clinical presentation

Data from Khoo BP, Leow YH. A review of inpatients with adverse drug reactions to allopurinol. Singapore Med J 2000;41:156–60.

Although HLA-B*5801 is most prevalent in East Asia, a study of European patients found a similar association.[38] HLA-B genotyping was performed on 150 patients enrolled in the European Study of Severe Cutaneous Adverse Reactions Registry (RegiSCAR). Even with an HLA-B*5801 frequency of 0.008 in the European population, the study found 31 patients with allopurinol-induced Stevens Johnson syndrome/toxic epidermal necrolysis or 61% carried the HLA-B*5801 allele. In contrast to the Hung and colleagues' study, the investigators concluded that HLA-B*5801 is a strong risk factor but neither sufficient nor necessary for the development of AHS. Whether HLA-B*5801 can be considered as a good marker for reducing the risk of AHS needs further analyses. As a result of the very low frequency of this allele in the non-Asian population, and the disease could be linked to other more prevalent and yet undetermined alleles in both populations, HLA testing is not currently recommended nor readily available in clinical practice.

Diuretics, such as hydrochlorothiazide and furosemide, have long been implicated as contributors to gout and hyperuricemia. Diuretics increase serum uric acid (SUA) levels by increasing UA reabsorption in the proximal tubule of the kidney. This effect occurs relatively quickly after the initiation of the diuretic and lasts throughout its use.[41] Diuretic use has been implicated in AHS and other ADRs as a result of decreased excretion of oxypurinol.[42,43] Understandably, if oxypurinol levels do contribute to ADRs, it would be prudent to minimize the levels. Clinically, one would expect the increase in oxypurinol levels caused by the diuretic to counter or eventually overcome the diuretic's hyperuricemic effect, yet this has been shown not to be the case.[44] This conundrum should cause the clinician to pause and evaluate the use of diuretics with allopurinol in patients, regardless of whether or not increases in oxypurinol occur.

In patients with renal insufficiency, it has been customary for clinicians to adjust or limit the maximum dose of allopurinol. Dose reduction in renal impairment is based on the reported relationship between "high-dose" allopurinol (>300 mg/d) in these patients and development of AHS.[42] Hande and colleagues[42] reported a case series of 6 patients with existing renal impairment in addition to 72 patients they found in a literature search, many of whom had existing renal impairment and were on diuretics as well. They concluded that AHS was caused by decreased renal clearance of oxypurinol, and therefore proposed renally adjusted dosing guidelines (**Table 3**). Based on their findings, Hande and colleagues[42] recommended that dosing should be modified to maintain oxypurinol levels between 20 and 100 µmol/L. Unfortunately, this dosing of allopurinol and level of oxypurinol may lead to undertreatment. A recent PD study found that to achieve an SUA lower than 6 mg/dL in at least 75% of subjects, serum oxypurinol levels higher than 100 µmol/L were required.[45] Additionally, no study has shown that dose reduction of allopurinol in CKD decreases the risk of AHS.

The proposed Hande and colleagues[42,46] guidelines have been widely recommended over the past 30 years, and even permeated clinical practice across specialties. Average prescribed daily dosages of allopurinol have been found to be 300 mg daily,[30] even in patients with normal renal function. The understandable fear of inducing AHS has led clinicians to have to choose between what is a perceived imbalanced risk of possible death to the patient and appropriately treating their chronic gout. Favorably balancing that scale, there have been reports of AHS occurring with "safe" oxypurinol levels (<100 µmol/L), whereas others with "unsafe" oxypurinol levels (>100 µmol/L) do not develop AHS.[47–49] More recent studies have convincingly shown that higher than recommended dosages of allopurinol do not predispose patients to AHS,[30,49] possibly antiquating Hande and colleagues' guidelines.

Stamp and colleagues[30] recently reported a retrospective case-control study of patients with gout, identifying 54 AHS cases and 157 controls matched for age, gender, diuretic use, and renal function. The analysis compared starting dose and dose at the time of the ADR between the cases and controls. The investigators found a strong and statistically significant relationship between the starting dose of allopurinol adjusted for estimated glomerular filtration rate (eGFR) and the risk of AHS. Cases were more likely to start on a higher than CrCL-based allopurinol dose compared with controls and controls were more likely to be commenced on lower than CrCL-based dose compared with cases. Additionally, they found that 91% of AHS cases and 36% of controls started on a dose of allopurinol at 1.5 mg or higher allopurinol per unit eGFR (mg/mL/min). The investigators concluded that allopurinol could be safely titrated as needed in patients, if the dose is started low enough and titrated slow enough (see **Table 3**).

Table 3
Proposed allopurinol dosing guidelines: old versus new

Hande et al,[42] 1984 Maximum Dosage Based on Renal Function		Stamp et al,[30] 2012 Starting Dosage Based on Renal Function	
Renal Function (mL/min)	Maximum Dosage	Starting Dosage	Renal Function (mg/mL/min)
0	100 mg 3 × per week	50 mg per week	<5
10	100 mg alternate days	50 mg twice per week	5–15
20	100 mg daily	50 mg every 2 d	16–30
40	150 mg daily	50 mg daily	31–45
60	200 mg daily	100 mg alternate days	46–60
100	300 mg daily	100 mg daily	61–90
		150 mg daily	91–130
		200 mg daily	>130

The underlying mechanism for AHS is not well understood, but is thought to be in part because of genetic susceptibility and cell-mediated immunity to allopurinol and oxypurinol, not necessarily the dose.[37,50] Although it is unclear how starting at lower doses of allopurinol may decrease the risk for significant reactions such AHS, it seems the "start low and go slow" mantra may not just help reduce the risk of acute flares, but also reduce the risk of AHS.

Febuxostat

Febuxostat is a nonpurine xanthine oxidase inhibitor that was approved in 2008 by the European Commission, and in February 2009 by the FDA. In contrast to allopurinol, the new ULT on the block has set doses. It is approved at 40 mg and 80 mg daily in the United States, and 120 mg in Europe. In a series of randomized trials, 40 mg and 80 mg were found to be noninferior and superior, respectively, to 300 mg of allopurinol.[51–53]

Febuxostat is a hepatically metabolized nonpurine analog, and although it shares with allopurinol an ability to inhibit xanthine oxidase, unlike allopurinol it does so by a noncompetitive mechanism. Febuxostat also differs from allopurinol in that it does not inhibit other enzymes in the pyramidine and purine synthetic and/or salvage pathways (such as purine nucleotide phosphorylase, hypoxanthine-guanine phosphoribosyltransferase, guanine deaminase, orotate phosphoribosyltransferase, or orotidine-5′-monophosphate decarboxylase).[54] Despite febuxostat being highly protein bound (99% albumin), many investigators have suggested that febuxostat's specificity may make it a safer alternative to currently available therapies, particularly with regard to drug-drug interactions, and patients with a history of allopurinol hypersensitivity.[51,55]

Drug-drug interactions

Febuxostat is relatively well tolerated with most medications and has a minimal drug-drug interaction profile (see **Table 1**). Because febuxostat has a highly bound state in plasma, investigators have examined drug-drug interactions between febuxostat and other highly protein-bound medications, such as captopril, digoxin, and warfarin.[56] Concomitant administration of febuxostat with these medications did not interfere or lead to toxic levels of any of the aforementioned medications.

As with allopurinol, febuxostat's ability to inhibit xanthine oxidase makes its use with medications metabolized by the same enzyme limited. Further speaking to its specificity and potentially stronger inhibition of xanthine oxidase compared with allopurinol (300 mg daily), febuxostat should be avoided in patients taking azathioprine or mercaptopurine.

Adverse drug reactions

In phase III trials, the incidence of adverse events among the 40 mg, 80 mg, and allopurinol groups were similar, with the exception of gout flares and liver enzyme elevations ($\geq$3 times the upper limit of normal). As a demonstration of febuxostat's ability to quickly lower SU levels, gout flares were one of the most common adverse events. Again, the risks of flares should be discussed with the patient, and prophylactic therapy should be initiated 1 to 2 weeks before initiating febuxostat (see **Table 2**).

Most adverse events were described as mild to moderate, including abnormal liver function tests, headaches, and diarrhea. Side effects occurring in fewer than 3% of the subjects included nausea and vomiting, neurologic signs and symptoms (dizziness, dysgeusia), fatigue, stomach discomfort, joint-related signs and symptoms (arthralgia, joint stiffness, swelling), and musculoskeletal/connective tissue signs and symptoms (back, chest wall, flank, stiffness, extremity pain). Across the phase III clinical trials, fewer than 1% of rashes were attributed to febuxostat, none of which were desquamating or life threatening.[53]

Analysis of liver enzyme elevations from pooled data indicated an increase of the event compared with allopurinol. Bilirubin levels did not exceed 2 mg/dL, and the elevation in liver enzymes did not appear to be dose related. Nevertheless, given the significant rates of obesity, metabolic syndrome, possible alcohol use, and chronic hepatitis, the investigators recommend periodic (not specified) liver function testing during treatment with both febuxostat and allopurinol (see **Table 2**).[53]

A potentially important distinction between febuxostat and allopurinol is their metabolism. As previously pointed out, allopurinol and its active metabolite, oxypurinol, are renally excreted, whereas febuxostat is hepatically metabolized. Despite accumulating evidence, allopurinol dosing in patients with renal impairment remains contentious. Phase III clinical trials have proven febuxostat to be safe in patients with moderate renal disease (serum Cr $\geq$1.6 but $\leq$2.0 mg/dL) in a small number of patients.[55] As many patients with gout have moderate or severe CKD, additional data are needed to ensure its safety in this population. A recent phase II trial using febuxostat in patients with an eGFR ranging from 15 to 50 mL/min has been completed.[57] The results from this study using 40 mg, 80 mg, and a 30-mg dose have yet to be reported.

Despite the growing evidence that renal insufficiency may not play a causative role in AHS, the patients with gout who have already experienced the potentially life-threatening syndrome need an alternative. Aside from desensitizing these patients or using uricosuric agents, which may not always be practical, gout treatment has been limited and frequently this group remains undertreated or untreated. In a series of 13 patients with a documented history of severe allopurinol reactions, 12 tolerated febuxostat.[58] One patient developed a hypersensitivity cutaneous vasculitis that was temporally related to febuxostat use. Although not definitive, the study provided evidence that the use of febuxostat may be safe in patients with sensitivity to allopurinol.

Knowing the association of CV disease and gout, medications that may increase the risk of CV disease events in such patients must be weighed carefully, regardless of the indication. In the 2 initial phase III trials, compared with placebo and allopurinol, there were a small number of CV deaths (6) in the febuxostat groups.[55] In response to the FDA's concerns regarding a potential CV signal, a 6-month, randomized, double-blinded, active-controlled trial was conducted. In the Confirmation of Febuxostat in Reducing and Maintaining Serum Urate Study (CONFIRMS) trial there were 2 deaths, neither were determined to be CV or febuxostat related. After review of the CONFIRMS data, the FDA concluded there was no definitive evidence of an increased risk for CV events with febuxostat.[59] The mixed results from the trial data require further clarity, and a long-term CV studies with febuxostat are needed and are currently under way.[60]

URATE OXIDASE
Pegloticase

Until recently, conventional gout therapies have fallen into 2 categories, oral xanthine oxidase inhibitors and oral uricosurics. Pegloticase was approved in September 2010 by the FDA for the treatment of hyperuricemia in patients with gout who have failed to normalize SU levels (<6 mg/dL) or continue to have signs and symptoms of gout on standard oral ULT.[61] The term refractory chronic gout (RCG) was given to patients who have severe, chronic gout who have failed or been intolerant to traditional ULTs.

Pegloticase is an intravenously (IV) administered recombinant mammalian urate oxidase (uricase) produced from a genetically modified *Escherichia coli* conjugated to multiple strands of monomethoxypoly ethyl glycol (PEG).[62] The attachment of what was once thought to be inert PEG, increases active uricase moiety's circulating half-life and decreases potential immunogenicity of the enzyme. Unlike other or ULT, pegloticase is unique in that it catalyzes the oxidation of uric acid into the more water-soluble allantoin, allowing for easier excretion by the kidney. The by-products of this lost process in humans and primates are the oxidative products, hydrogen peroxide and carbon dioxide.[63] Owing to the production of hydrogen peroxide and risk of hemolysis or methemoglobinemia, the one definitive contraindication to pegloticase are patients with a glucose-6-phosphate dehydrogenase deficiency (see **Table 2**). The structure, metabolism, and IV administration of pegloticase make its safety profile unlike other available oral ULTs.

Drug-drug interaction
To date there have been no formal studies of pegloticase-drug interactions (see **Table 1**). It has been found that the efficacy and potential reactions to pegloticase correlate with the development of antibodies to the PEGylated portion of the medication. It has been suggested that these anti-PEG antibodies (immunoglobulin [Ig]G and IgM) could potentially bind to other PEGylated products and interfere with their efficacy. The impact of anti-PEG antibodies to pegloticase on other PEG-containing therapeutics has not been studied and is still unknown.

The concomitant use of other ULTs with pegloticase is not an interaction, but a confounder. When treating with pegloticase, monitoring the SU levels before the second and subsequent infusion is essential to prevent ADRs (see the following section). Therefore, its use with other ULTs may result in an additive hypouricemic effect and is not recommended.

Adverse drug reactions
There were 2 replicate, multicenter, randomized, double-blind, placebo-controlled phase III trials for pegloticase. Two hundred twenty-five patients were randomized to pegloticase every 4 weeks, pegloticose every 2 weeks, or placebo. Baseline characteristics were similar across the 212 intent-to-treat patients enrolled.[64] Mean disease duration of the study population was 15 years, with an average of 10 flares during in the prior 18 months.[61] *Responders* to the medication were considered those who maintained a plasma urate level lower than 6.0 mg/dL at least 80% of the time during the 6-month trial.[64] *Nonresponders* were considered those who did not meet the responder criteria or who did not complete the trial.

Impressively, enrollment was inclusive and included "real-world" patients who had multiple comorbidities. Metabolic, renal disorders, and CV comorbidities or risk factors were present in more than 80% of study participants.[64] Highlighting the enzymatic action of pegloticose, there was no evidence in any of the clinical trials that dose adjustment or caution should be taken in patients with hepatic disease or CKD. That said, owing to potential infusion reactions (IR), the necessity to premedicate patients before every infusion with corticosteroids, antihistamines, and acetaminophen may have an impact on patients with comborbid conditions (see **Table 2**). For example, premedicating patients with heart failure with corticosteroids (causing water retention) and then infusing fluids may overload them if their heart failure is not well compensated.

The doses of steroids before every 2-week infusion are considered high, and range from 200 mg of hydrocortisone sodium succinate (Solu-Cortef) as used in the clinical trials, to 125 mg of methylprednisolone sodium succinate (Solu-Medrol) used in practice in patients without diabetes mellitus or severe heart failure. Corticosteroids come with an array of additional risks when given as a bolus, but it is necessary to point out that, when averaged over the course of 6 months, the dose would equal 14 mg and 8 mg of hydrocortisone and methylprednisolone, respectively. Still a considerable dose, the amount of preinfusion corticosteroids has been successfully reduced in patients who have been deemed responders (data not published).

Pelgoticase rapidly decreases SU levels, and, as expected, the most common adverse events were gout flares despite prophylaxis with colchicines or NSAIDs. The next most common adverse events were IRs.[64] The most common signs and symptoms of an IR include erythema, urticaria, dyspnea, flushing, chest discomfort, chest pain, and rash.

Serious IRs occurred in 5% and 8% of the pegloticase biweekly and monthly, respectively.[64] Resolution of all IRs began within minutes and resolved quickly after slowing or discontinuing the infusion or initiating supportive treatment (epinephrine was used in 1 patient).[64] In a retrospective analysis of IRs, 5 patients experienced IRs with signs and symptoms that met criteria for anaphylaxis from the National Institute of Allergy and Infectious Disease/Food Allergy and Anaphylaxis Network.[64,65] These included 2 patients each in the pegloticase biweekly and pegloticase monthly cohort and 1 patient who experienced these clinical features during the first infusion. All of these reactions were judged as mild to moderate in severity by the investigator.[64]

The immunogenicity of a medication typically correlates with ADRs, such as infusion reactions and anaphylaxis. Approximately 20% of the patients enrolled in the phase III trials had positive anti-PEG antibodies before their first infusion and raise the possibility that PEG products are not as inert as once thought. Not necessarily correlating with preexisting PEG antibodies, antibodies to pegloticase (anti-PEG IgM and IgG) developed relatively quickly and developed in 89% of the pegloticase cohort at various titers.[64]

The use of pegloticase and IRs has been a concern and has precluded its use for many clinicians. Finding ways to avoid or prevent reactions has been and remains a priority for investigators. Fortunately, ways have been found to reduce such risks. A post hoc analysis of the phase III trials found IRs were reported in 60% of patients with anti-PEG antibodies titers greater than 1:2430 compared with 19% in whom titers never exceeded 1:2430. More importantly, the investigators found the loss of urate-lowering efficacy (urate >6.0 mg/dL) preceded the first IR in 91% of patients receiving biweekly pegloticase and 71% receiving monthly pegloticase.[64]

The investigators concluded SU levels could be used as a surrogate for high antibody production. Therefore, monitoring SU levels within 24 to 48 hours (I prefer <24 hours given the variability in the drug's half-life from patient to patient and from first dose to last dose, ranging from 7.5–16.8 days and 3.9–39.2 days, respectively[66]) is a safety siren, so to speak, for preventing infusion and anaphylactic reactions. When using pegloticase, it is recommended that providers monitor SU level before the second and subsequent infusions, and consider discontinuing treatment if levels increase to above 6 mg/dL, particularly when 2 consecutive levels higher than 6 mg/dL are observed.[61] Most responders maintain serum urate levels lower than 2.0 mg/dL, and the nonresponders typically declare themselves quickly within the first 2 to 3 months of therapy. Using oral ULT with pegloticase is not necessary, and may result in an additive effect, giving the provider a false sense of security and inability to accurately determine pegloticase's effect on SU levels (see **Table 2**).

The decision to discontinue the infusions after the first versus after the second SU above 6 mg/dL must be made on a case-by-case basis. Some patients will eventually respond after the first SU higher than 6 mg/dL. Therefore, the provider must take into account how the patient tolerated the previous infusion; the patient's comorbidities, quality of life, and disability from chronic gout; and other treatment options or limitations to treatment they may have before discontinuing the medication.

In the phase III trials, 18% of the study patients had known coronary artery disease.[61] There were 2 deaths reported during the treatment period attributed to CV disease, and 1 nonfatal myocardial infarction. In the pegloticase treatment group, 12% of the patients treated had a history of heart failure.[61] There were 2 cases with preexisting heart failure that had an exacerbation during the trial. In addition, during the open-label extension study, 4 patients experienced exacerbation of preexisting heart failure.[61] The incidence of CV events in patients with known CV disease, underscores the need for long-term data in this population. It is likely the premedication regimen and fluid bolus for patients with heart failure may actually make a greater impact than pegloticase itself. Clinical experience with this medication is still in its infancy, and further studies are needed to critically assess its risks in patients with CV and those with other comorbidities. An open-labeled, long-term extension trial to address such questions is ongoing.

URICOSURICS
Probenecid

Although allopurinol is the ULT of choice in chronic gout, uricosuric agents, such as probenecid, sulfinpyrazone (Anturane), and benzbromarone, were introduced for the treatment of gout before allopurinol.[67] Because benzbromarone was withdrawn from the market by the original manufacturer owing to potential hepatotoxicity, and the availability of sulfinpyrazone is limited, probenecid is the only uricosuric readily available in the United States to date. Initially developed for inhibiting the renal tubular secretion of penicillin in the mid-1940s, probenecid was discovered around 1950 to be a uricosuric and beneficial in lowering SU in patients with gout.[68] The medication is extensively metabolized by glucuronide conjugation and oxidation of the alkyl side chains, and the half-life in plasma is dose dependent (4–12 hours).[69]

Drug-drug interactions

Probenecid and its metabolites are primarily bound to albumin and most of the drug-drug interactions are attributable to its ability block the transport of acidic drugs across transporters in the kidney.[69] Importantly, all NSAIDs, particularly ketorolac, should be used with caution, as renal excretion is markedly decreased (see **Table 1**).

Adverse drug reactions

Studies in patients with and without gout have revealed that rash is the most common ADR leading to discontinuation.[68,70] Additional ADRs in patients with gout include gastrointestinal, dizziness, fatigue, headache, flushing, muscle pain or cramps, and, of course, gout flares. Probenecid should be used cautiously in patients with a history of renal calculi and those with normal or increased excretion of uric acid (overproducers) (see **Table 2**).[23] To minimize the risk of gout flares and renal calculi, the recommended dosage is 250 mg twice daily for 1 week, followed by 500 mg twice daily, with a maximum dosage of 2000 mg daily.[71,72] In patients with renal impairment, it may be beneficial to titrate the dose slower, increasing by 500 mg every 4 weeks and not exceeding 2000 mg daily.[71] The risk of nephrolithiasis can be further reduced by maintenance of a high urine volume (>2 L/d) and alkalization of urine.[72]

In clinical practice, probenecid has been thought to be ineffective in the setting of renal insufficiency (CrCl <50 mL/min); however, in a small observational study, it was found to be well tolerated and beneficial in achieving target SU levels when used in combination with allopurinol in patients with renal insufficiency.[26] Despite the declining use in the United States and abroad,[73] probenecid in patients with gout is generally well tolerated, and it still may be a beneficial and safe therapeutic option in patients intolerant to xanthine oxidase inhibitors or in combination in patients whose SU targets have not been achieved.

SUMMARY

Gout is the most common inflammatory arthropathy, and many patients with gout are inadequately treated. The undertreatment of such a treatable disease has in part been because of a lack of understanding and fear of potential adverse effects of traditional therapies used to lower SU levels. Comorbidities commonly associated with gout can impede treatment and turn a straightforward disease into a conundrum. Changing dogma in medicine may take a few decades, but the development of new therapies to treat this ancient disease has rejuvenated dialogue and awareness among patients, primary care providers, and rheumatologists.

The discourse has not been only about new ULTs, but also of the old. Recently published data regarding allopurinol dosing and potential ADRs provide a step toward reeducating clinicians and their perceptions of how to safely treat patients with gout with and without the comorbidities that so often accompany it. More specific and targeted treatment options, such as febuxostat and pegloticase, have given clinicians additional opportunities to effectively treat chronic gout, resolve their urate burden, and decrease associated morbidity. Additional safety concerns arise beyond signals seen during clinical trials as a new medication is used in day-to-day practice, but as the clinician's understanding of a novel therapy evolves, so does the ability to avert potential safety risks so as to provide the patient with the most benefit.

REFERENCES

1. Zhu Y, Pandya BJ, Choi HK. Prevalence of gout and hyperuricemia in the US general population: the National Health and Nutrition Examination Survey 2007-2008. Arthritis Rheum 2011;63:3136–41.
2. Arromdee E, Michet CJ, Crowson CS, et al. Epidemiology of gout: is the incidence rising? J Rheumatol 2002;29:2403–6.
3. Weaver AL. Epidemiology of gout. Cleve Clin J Med 2008;75(Suppl 5):S9–12.
4. Driver JA, Djousse L, Logroscino G, et al. Incidence of cardiovascular disease and cancer in advanced age: prospective cohort study. BMJ 2008;337:a2467.
5. Folsom AR, Yatsuya H, Nettleton JA, et al. Community prevalence of ideal cardiovascular health, by the American Heart Association definition, and relationship with cardiovascular disease incidence. J Am Coll Cardiol 2011;57:1690–6.
6. Choi HK, Atkinson K, Karlson EW, et al. Obesity, weight change, hypertension, diuretic use, and risk of gout in men: the health professionals follow-up study. Arch Intern Med 2005;165:742–8.
7. Choi HK, Curhan G. Independent impact of gout on mortality and risk for coronary heart disease. Circulation 2007;116:894–900.
8. Pillinger MH, Goldfarb DS, Keenan RT. Gout and its comorbidities. Bull NYU Hosp Jt Dis 2010;68:199–203.
9. Keenan RT, O'Brien WR, Lee KH, et al. Prevalence of contraindications and prescription of pharmacologic therapies for gout. Am J Med 2011;124:155–63.
10. Zhu Y, Pandya BJ, Choi HK. Comorbidities of gout and hyperuricemia in the US general population: NHANES 2007-2008. Am J Med 2012;125(7):679–687.e1.

11. Mikuls TR, Farrar JT, Bilker WB, et al. Gout epidemiology: results from the UK General Practice Research Database, 1990-1999. Ann Rheum Dis 2005;64: 267–72.

12. Riedel AA, Nelson M, Wallace K, et al. Prevalence of comorbid conditions and prescription medication use among patients with gout and hyperuricemia in a managed care setting. J Clin Rheumatol 2004;10:308–14.

13. Wyngaarden JB, Rundles RW, Metz EN. Allopurinol in the treatment of gout. Ann Intern Med 1965;62:842–7.

14. Talbott JH, Bishop C, Norcross BM, et al. The clinical and metabolic effects of benemid in patients with gout. Trans Assoc Am Physicians 1951;64:372–7.

15. Sarawate CA, Patel PA, Schumacher HR, et al. Serum urate levels and gout flares: analysis from managed care data. J Clin Rheumatol 2006;12:61–5.

16. Mikuls TR, Curtis JR, Allison JJ, et al. Medication errors with the use of allopurinol and colchicine: a retrospective study of a national, anonymous Internet-accessible error reporting system. J Rheumatol 2006;33:562–6.

17. Mikuls TR, Farrar JT, Bilker WB, et al. Suboptimal physician adherence to quality indicators for the management of gout and asymptomatic hyperuricaemia: results from the UK General Practice Research Database (GPRD). Rheumatology (Oxford) 2005;44:1038–42.

18. Sarawate CA, Brewer KK, Yang W, et al. Gout medication treatment patterns and adherence to standards of care from a managed care perspective. Mayo Clin Proc 2006;81:925–34.

19. Perez-Ruiz F, Calabozo M, Pijoan JI, et al. Effect of urate-lowering therapy on the velocity of size reduction of tophi in chronic gout. Arthritis Rheum 2002;47: 356–60.

20. Dal Pan GJ. Communicating the risks of medicine: time to move forward. Med Care 2012;50:463–5.

21. Kongkaew C, Noyce PR, Ashcroft DM. Hospital admissions associated with adverse drug reactions: a systematic review of prospective observational studies. Ann Pharmacother 2008;42:1017–25.

22. Khanna PP, Perez-Ruiz F, Maranian P, et al. Long-term therapy for chronic gout results in clinically important improvements in the health-related quality of life: short form-36 is responsive to change in chronic gout. Rheumatology (Oxford) 2011;50:740–5.

23. Schlesinger N. Difficult-to-treat gouty arthritis: a disease warranting better management. Drugs 2011;71:1413–39.

24. Wu EQ, Forsythe A, Guerin A, et al. Comorbidity burden, healthcare resource utilization, and costs in chronic gout patients refractory to conventional urate-lowering therapy. Am J Ther 2011. [Epub ahead of print].

25. Pacher P, Nivorozhkin A, Szabo C. Therapeutic effects of xanthine oxidase inhibitors: renaissance half a century after the discovery of allopurinol. Pharmacol Rev 2006;58:87–114.

26. Stocker SL, Graham GG, McLachlan AJ, et al. Pharmacokinetic and pharmacodynamic interaction between allopurinol and probenecid in patients with gout. J Rheumatol 2011;38:904–10.

27. Pennell DJ, Nunan TO, O'Doherty MJ, et al. Fatal Stevens-Johnson syndrome in a patient on captopril and allopurinol. Lancet 1984;1:463.

28. Samanta A, Burden AC. Fever, myalgia, and arthralgia in a patient on captopril and allopurinol. Lancet 1984;1:679.

29. Ahmad S. Allopurinol and enalapril. Drug induced anaphylactic coronary spasm and acute myocardial infarction. Chest 1995;108:586.

30. Stamp LK, Taylor WJ, Jones PB, et al. Starting dose is a risk factor for allopurinol hypersensitivity syndrome: a proposed safe starting dose of allopurinol. Arthritis Rheum 2012;64(8):2529–36.
31. Khanna D, Fuldeore MJ, Meissner BL, et al. The incidence of allopurinol hypersensitivity syndrome: a population perspective. Arthritis Rheum 2008;60:S542.
32. Lang PG Jr. Severe hypersensitivity reactions to allopurinol. South Med J 1979; 72:1361–8.
33. Tassaneeyakul W, Jantararoungtong T, Chen P, et al. Strong association between HLA-B*5801 and allopurinol-induced Stevens-Johnson syndrome and toxic epidermal necrolysis in a Thai population. Pharmacogenet Genomics 2009;19:704–9.
34. Dalbeth N, Stamp L. Allopurinol dosing in renal impairment: walking the tightrope between adequate urate lowering and adverse events. Semin Dial 2007;20:391–5.
35. Lee HY, Ariyasinghe JT, Thirumoorthy T. Allopurinol hypersensitivity syndrome: a preventable severe cutaneous adverse reaction? Singapore Med J 2008;49: 384–7.
36. Turnheim K, Krivanek P, Oberbauer R. Pharmacokinetics and pharmacodynamics of allopurinol in elderly and young subjects. Br J Clin Pharmacol 1999;48:501–9.
37. Hung SI, Chung WH, Liou LB, et al. HLA-B*5801 allele as a genetic marker for severe cutaneous adverse reactions caused by allopurinol. Proc Natl Acad Sci U S A 2005;102:4134–9.
38. Lonjou C, Borot N, Sekula P, et al. A European study of HLA-B in Stevens-Johnson syndrome and toxic epidermal necrolysis related to five high-risk drugs. Pharmacogenet Genomics 2008;18:99–107.
39. Kaniwa N, Saito Y, Aihara M, et al. HLA-B locus in Japanese patients with anti-epileptics and allopurinol-related Stevens-Johnson syndrome and toxic epidermal necrolysis. Pharmacogenomics 2008;9:1617–22.
40. Kang HR, Jee YK, Kim YS, et al. Positive and negative associations of HLA class I alleles with allopurinol-induced SCARs in Koreans. Pharmacogenet Genomics 2011;21:303–7.
41. Reyes AJ. Cardiovascular drugs and serum uric acid. Cardiovasc Drugs Ther 2003;17:397–414.
42. Hande KR, Noone RM, Stone WJ. Severe allopurinol toxicity. Description and guidelines for prevention in patients with renal insufficiency. Am J Med 1984;76:47–56.
43. Yamamoto T, Moriwaki Y, Takahashi S, et al. Effect of furosemide on renal excretion of oxypurinol and purine bases. Metabolism 2001;50:241–5.
44. Stamp LK, Barclay ML, O'Donnell JL, et al. Furosemide increases plasma oxypurinol without lowering serum urate—a complex drug interaction: implications for clinical practice. Rheumatology (Oxford) 2012;51(9):1670–6.
45. Stamp LK, Barclay ML, O'Donnell JL, et al. Relationship between serum urate and plasma oxypurinol in the management of gout: determination of minimum plasma oxypurinol concentration to achieve a target serum urate level. Clin Pharmacol Ther 2011;90:392–8.
46. Emmerson BT. The management of gout. N Engl J Med 1996;334:445–51.
47. Emmerson BT, Gordon RB, Cross M, et al. Plasma oxipurinol concentrations during allopurinol therapy. Br J Rheumatol 1987;26:445–9.
48. Dalbeth N, Kumar S, Stamp L, et al. Dose adjustment of allopurinol according to creatinine clearance does not provide adequate control of hyperuricemia in patients with gout. J Rheumatol 2006;33:1646–50.
49. Vazquez-Mellado J, Morales EM, Pacheco-Tena C, et al. Relation between adverse events associated with allopurinol and renal function in patients with gout. Ann Rheum Dis 2001;60:981–3.

50. Emmerson BT, Hazelton RA, Frazer IH. Some adverse reactions to allopurinol may be mediated by lymphocyte reactivity to oxypurinol. Arthritis Rheum 1988; 31:436–40.

51. Becker MA, Schumacher HR Jr, Wortmann RL, et al. Febuxostat compared with allopurinol in patients with hyperuricemia and gout. N Engl J Med 2005;353: 2450–61.

52. Schumacher HR Jr, Becker MA, Wortmann RL, et al. Effects of febuxostat versus allopurinol and placebo in reducing serum urate in subjects with hyperuricemia and gout: a 28-week, phase III, randomized, double-blind, parallel-group trial. Arthritis Rheum 2008;59:1540–8.

53. Becker MA, Schumacher HR, Espinoza LR, et al. The urate-lowering efficacy and safety of febuxostat in the treatment of the hyperuricemia of gout: the CONFIRMS trial. Arthritis Res Ther 2010;12:R63.

54. Takano Y, Hase-Aoki K, Horiuchi H, et al. Selectivity of febuxostat, a novel non-purine inhibitor of xanthine oxidase/xanthine dehydrogenase. Life Sci 2005;76:1835–47.

55. Keenan RT, Pillinger MH. Febuxostat: a new agent for lowering serum urate. Drugs Today (Barc) 2009;45:247–60.

56. Mukoyoshi M, Nishimura S, Hoshide S, et al. In vitro drug-drug interaction studies with febuxostat, a novel non-purine selective inhibitor of xanthine oxidase: plasma protein binding, identification of metabolic enzymes and cytochrome P450 inhibition. Xenobiotica 2008;38:496–510.

57. Effect of febuxostat on renal function in patients with gout and moderate to severe renal impairment. 2012. Available at: http://clinicaltrials.gov/ct2/show/NCT01 082640?term=febuxostat&rank=4. Accessed July 30, 2012.

58. Chohan S. Safety and efficacy of febuxostat treatment in subjects with gout and severe allopurinol adverse reactions. J Rheumatol 2011;38:1957–9.

59. Ernst ME, Fravel MA. Febuxostat: a selective xanthine-oxidase/xanthine-dehydrogenase inhibitor for the management of hyperuricemia in adults with gout. Clin Ther 2009;31:2503–18.

60. White WB, Grady D, Giudice LC, et al. A cardiovascular safety study of LibiGel (testosterone gel) in postmenopausal women with elevated cardiovascular risk and hypoactive sexual desire disorder. Am Heart J 2012;163:27–32.

61. Krystexxa (pegloticase): prescribing information. East Brunswick (NJ): Savient Pharmaceuticals, Inc; 2012.

62. Sundy JS, Ganson NJ, Kelly SJ, et al. Pharmacokinetics and pharmacodynamics of intravenous PEGylated recombinant mammalian urate oxidase in patients with refractory gout. Arthritis Rheum 2007;56:1021–8.

63. Hershfield MS, Roberts LJ 2nd, Ganson NJ, et al. Treating gout with pegloticase, a PEGylated urate oxidase, provides insight into the importance of uric acid as an antioxidant in vivo. Proc Natl Acad Sci U S A 2010;107:14351–6.

64. Sundy JS, Baraf HS, Yood RA, et al. Efficacy and tolerability of pegloticase for the treatment of chronic gout in patients refractory to conventional treatment: two randomized controlled trials. JAMA 2011;306:711–20.

65. Sampson HA, Munoz-Furlong A, Campbell RL, et al. Second symposium on the definition and management of anaphylaxis: summary report—second National Institute of Allergy and Infectious Disease/Food Allergy and Anaphylaxis Network symposium. Ann Emerg Med 2006;47:373–80.

66. Sundy JS, Becker MA, Baraf HS, et al. Reduction of plasma urate levels following treatment with multiple doses of pegloticase (polyethylene glycol-conjugated uricase) in patients with treatment-failure gout: results of a phase II randomized study. Arthritis Rheum 2008;58:2882–91.

67. Zhang W, Doherty M, Bardin T, et al. EULAR evidence based recommendations for gout. Part II: management. Report of a task force of the EULAR Standing Committee for International Clinical Studies Including Therapeutics (ESCISIT). Ann Rheum Dis 2006;65:1312–24.
68. Boger WP, Strickland SC. Probenecid (benemid); its uses and side-effects in 2,502 patients. AMA Arch Intern Med 1955;95:83–92.
69. Cunningham RF, Israili ZH, Dayton PG. Clinical pharmacokinetics of probenecid. Clin Pharm 1981;6:135–51.
70. Reinders MK, van Roon EN, Jansen TL, et al. Efficacy and tolerability of urate-lowering drugs in gout: a randomised controlled trial of benzbromarone versus probenecid after failure of allopurinol. Ann Rheum Dis 2009;68:51–6.
71. Probenecid prescribing information. 2012. Available at: http://dailymed.nlm.nih.gov/dailymed/lookup.cfm?setid=5ca3dd4c-b8b4-4131-a066-214dabb2576f#nlm 34067-9. Accessed June 23, 2012.
72. Fam AG. Gout in the elderly. Clinical presentation and treatment. Drugs Aging 1998;13:229–43.
73. Robbins N, Koch SE, Tranter M, et al. The history and future of probenecid. Cardiovasc Toxicol 2012;12:1–9.
74. Allopurinol: drug information: Lexicomp; 2006. Available at: http://www.uptodate.com/crlsql/interact/frameset.jsp. Accessed July 29, 2012.
75. Uloric (febuxostat): prescribing information. Deerfield (IL): Takeda Pharmaceuticals American, Inc; 2011.

Safety of Bisphosphonates

Catalina Orozco, MD[a], Naim M. Maalouf, MD[b],*

KEYWORDS

- Bisphosphonate • Safety • Side effects • Osteonecrosis of the jaw
- Atypical femoral fracture • Atrial fibrillation • Esophageal cancer • Esophagitis

KEY POINTS

- Although placebo-controlled clinical trials lasting 3 to 4 years have shown that bisphosphonates significantly reduce the risk of osteoporotic fractures, limited data are available on their antifracture efficacy beyond 5 years of therapy.
- Common side effects of bisphosphonates include upper gastrointestinal tract irritation with oral bisphosphonates and an acute phase response with intravenous bisphosphonates.
- Osteonecrosis of the jaw and atypical femoral fractures have emerged as rare complications associated with long-term bisphosphonate use, and the incidence of these complications may increase with duration of bisphosphonate exposure.
- The association of bisphosphonate therapy with esophageal cancer and atrial fibrillation is not well substantiated.
- Necessity of continued bisphosphonate therapy should be periodically reassessed after 5 years of therapy in patients with osteoporosis.

INTRODUCTION

Bisphosphonates are antiresorptive medications that reduce osteoclastic activity, resulting in decreased bone turnover, improved bone mineral density, and reduced risk of osteoporotic fractures. As of 2008, bisphosphonates were used by more than 5.1 million patients in the United States alone, with a prevalence of approximately 12% among women older than 55 years.[1] Although overall well-tolerated in large-scale osteoporosis clinical trials, several adverse events have been reported with their use in clinical trials and in the postmarketing era. This article discusses the safety of bisphosphonates for the treatment of osteoporosis, identifies at-risk populations for these side effects, and provides guidance for their use.

[a] Rheumatology Associates, 8144 Walnut Hill Lane, Suite 800, Dallas, TX 75231, USA;
[b] Department of Internal Medicine, Center for Mineral Metabolism and Clinical Research, University of Texas Southwestern Medical Center, 5323 Harry Hines Boulevard, Dallas, TX 75390-8885, USA
* Corresponding author.
E-mail address: naim.maalouf@utsouthwestern.edu

Rheum Dis Clin N Am 38 (2012) 681–705
http://dx.doi.org/10.1016/j.rdc.2012.09.001
0889-857X/12/$ – see front matter © 2012 Elsevier Inc. All rights reserved.
rheumatic.theclinics.com

PHARMACOLOGY OF BISPHOSPHONATES
Mechanism of Action

Bisphosphonates consist of a group of compounds with a common phosphorus-carbon-phosphorus backbone that resembles the phosphorus-oxygen-phosphorus structure of native pyrophosphate,[2] and different side chains that are specific to each compound. Their major pharmacologic property is inhibition of bone resorption, which is achieved through (1) strong attachment to the hydroxyapatite mineral found in bone, (2) uptake by osteoclasts resorbing bone, and (3) inhibition of osteoclast function or induction of osteoclast apoptosis.[2,3] Reduced bone resorption results in improvement in bone mineral density and reduction in fracture rates. Bisphosphonates secondarily reduce bone formation due to the normal "coupling" between bone resorption and bone formation that occurs at individual resorption units.

Pharmacokinetics

Because of their high affinity to hydroxyapatite, bisphosphonates exhibit unique pharmacokinetic properties: after the ingestion of an oral bisphosphonate, less than 1% of the drug is absorbed from the gastrointestinal tract, whereas intravenous bisphosphonates are injected directly into the circulation. Of the fraction that reaches the circulation, approximately 50% is excreted unmetabolized in the urine, and the remaining 50% is taken up avidly in the skeleton, with little uptake by other tissues. Thereafter, bisphosphonates are slowly released back into circulation after uptake by osteoclasts at the surface of bone, and a much slower elimination phase is seen, with an estimated mean terminal half-life of greater than 10 years.[4]

Pharmacology of Different Bisphosphonates

The mechanism through which osteoclast dysfunction occurs differs between nitrogen-containing bisphosphonates and non–nitrogen-containing bisphosphonates, or simple bisphosphonates. The nitrogen-containing bisphosphonate group (which includes alendronate, ibandronate, risedronate, and zoledronic acid [ZA]) exerts its effects through inhibiting the enzyme farnesyl pyrophosphate synthase (FFP synthase) that prevents the prenylation of small GTPases, thus reducing osteoclast activity. On the other hand, simple bisphosphonates (etidronate, clodronate, and tiludronate) are metabolized in the osteoclast cytosol to ATP analogs that induce osteoclast apoptosis.[5] Even among the widely used nitrogen-containing bisphosphonates, the potency of individual bisphosphonates is further determined by the degree of affinity to hydroxyapatite and the extent of inhibition of FFP synthase.

EFFICACY OF BISPHOSPHONATES

Currently 4 bisphosphonates are approved by the U.S. Food and Drug Administration (FDA) for the treatment of osteoporosis in the United States: alendronate, ibandronate, risedronate, and ZA. All 4 medications have been shown in FDA registration trials[6–9] to reduce the risk for vertebral fractures over a 3-year period. In these trials, some of these medications also significantly reduced hip fractures (alendronate and ZA) and nonvertebral fractures (risedronate and ZA).[6,8,10] In addition to the FDA registration trials, data from nonregistration trials and pooled or observational data have supported a reduced rate of vertebral, nonvertebral, and hip fractures for all 4 agents.[11–14] Overall, point estimates of relative vertebral fracture risk reduction range from 40% to 70%, and relative hip fracture reduction ranges from 40% to 50% with these drugs. This relative reduction risk for fractures seems to only be partly explained by improvement in bone mineral density, as evidenced by the nonlinear relationship between bone density and fracture reduction.[15,16]

The optimal duration of bisphosphonate therapy in patients with osteoporosis is unknown. Data from extension arms of the larger clinical trials with alendronate, risedronate, and ZA suggest that alendronate therapy beyond 5 years does not significantly decrease the risk for fractures, except for clinically recognized vertebral fractures.[17] Furthermore, post hoc analysis of the same data revealed that nonvertebral fractures were reduced in patients treated for 10 years (vs 5 years) with alendronate only if femoral neck T-scores remained below –2.5 after 5 years of therapy or if they had already sustained a vertebral fracture.[18] In the extension trial for ZA comparing 3 versus 6 years of therapy, similar effects were seen, with significant reduction in vertebral fractures and no difference in nonvertebral fracture risk.[19] Eastell and colleagues[20] reported the results of stopping risedronate therapy in patients treated for either 2 or 7 years. Risedronate discontinuation for 1 year led to increases in the levels of markers of bone turnover in both groups toward baseline and decreases in total hip bone mineral density, whereas lumbar spine and femoral neck bone mineral density remained unchanged. Data from extension trials is limited by the group of patients included, which may have led to selection bias, and by the trial design, which may be underpowered for fracture reduction. However, overall the available data suggest that bisphosphonate treatment beyond 5 years leads to further increases in bone mineral density at the spine but not at other sites, and only a reduction of vertebral fractures and nonvertebral fractures in high-risk patients (those with prior vertebral fractures or T-scores below –2.5 after 5 years of therapy). Long-term studies to evaluate fracture risk are unlikely to be further undertaken.

SAFETY OF BISPHOSPHONATES
Atypical Femoral Fractures

Bisphosphonate therapy has been shown in clinical trials to significantly decrease the rates of hip fractures in patients with osteoporosis.[10,21–23] In 2005, a report was published describing patients treated long-term with oral bisphosphonates who developed unusual low-trauma fractures, often involving the femoral shafts.[24] In subsequent years, a growing number of case reports and series were published citing an increased risk for atypical femoral fractures (AFFs) in patients treated with prolonged bisphosphonate therapy.[25–29] This finding prompted the American Society for Bone and Mineral Research to convene a multidisciplinary task force, which published its findings on AFFs in a report in the fall of 2010,[30] providing a definition of these fractures (**Table 1**). The report stated that a causal link between AFFs and bisphosphonate use could not be established, but that a potential association with prolonged bisphosphonate use was noted.[30] Shortly afterward, the FDA required a label change for oral bisphosphonates, describing the uncertainty regarding the optimal duration of bisphosphonate use for the treatment or prevention of osteoporosis.

Unlike the more prevalent osteoporotic femoral neck (**Fig. 1**A) and intertrochanteric fractures, AFFs are commonly located in the upper third of the femur but distal to the lesser trochanter.[30] They may occur with minimal or no trauma, and be preceded by thigh or groin pain. Unlike the typical femoral shaft fractures (see **Fig. 1**B), AFFs have distinctive radiographic features, including a transverse or short oblique configuration, and are noncomminuted (see **Fig. 1**C). Complete fractures (see **Fig. 1**C) extend through both cortices and may have a medial spike, whereas incomplete fractures (see **Fig. 1**D) compromise only the lateral cortex. Other features that may be present include a localized periosteal reaction, increased cortical thickness, and delayed healing. AFFs may be bilateral in almost 50% of patients.[30]

Table 1
Features of atypical femoral fractures[a]

Major Features[b]	Minor Features[b]
Location between the lesser trochanter and the supracondylar flare	Generalized increased cortical thickness of the diaphysis
Occurs with minimal or no trauma	Delayed healing
Transverse or short oblique configuration	Prodromal symptoms: pain in the groin/thigh
Noncomminuted	Bilateral fractures and symptoms
May be incomplete (involving only the lateral cortex) or complete (extending through both cortices)	Localized periosteal reaction of the lateral cortex
	Comorbid conditions: rheumatoid arthritis, vitamin D deficiency, hypophosphatasia Use of pharmaceutical agents (eg, glucocorticoids, bisphosphonates, proton pump inhibitors)

[a] According to Report on atypical subtrochanteric and diaphyseal femoral fractures from Task Force of the American Society for Bone and Mineral Research. J Bone Miner Res 2010;25(11):2267–94.
[b] All major features are required to satisfy the case definition of an AFF. None of the minor features are required but some have been associated with these fractures.

The true incidence of this condition is not known, although recent publications have examined this question. Dell and colleagues[31] reported that the incidence of AFF in a group of 1.8 million older patients enrolled at Kaiser Southern California gradually increased from 1.78 per 100,000 person-years in patients receiving bisphosphonates

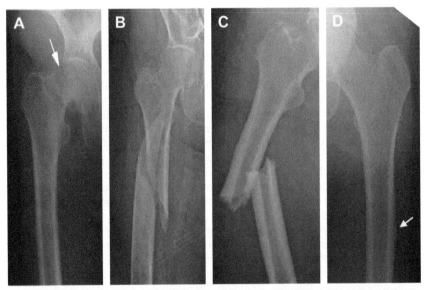

Fig. 1. Sites of femur fractures. (*A*) Femoral neck fracture. (*B*) Typical femoral shaft fracture. (*C*) Complete atypical femoral shaft fracture. (*D*) Incomplete atypical femoral shaft fracture. ([*B, C*] *Adapted from* Lenart BA. Association of low-energy femoral fractures with prolonged bisphosphonate use: a case control study. Osteoporos Int 2009;20:1353–62; with permission; and [*D*] *From* Compston J. Pathophysiology of atypical femoral fractures and osteonecrosis of the jaw. Osteoporos Int 2011;22:2951–61; with permission.)

for less than 2 years to 113.1 per 100,000 person-years in patients receiving therapy for 8.0 to 9.9 years (**Fig. 2**). In a separate study from a single center, the incidence rate of AFF was low (3.2 cases per 100,000 person-years) and on average increased by 10.7% per year in patients receiving bisphosphonate therapy. Although these data do not prove a causal association between bisphosphonate use and AFF, the rising risk with increasing bisphosphonate exposure supports this association.

At the same time, the incidence of AFF seems to be rare compared with the incidence of osteoporotic hip (femoral neck) fractures. In the study by Dell and colleagues,[31] the incidence of the more typical hip fractures was significantly higher than that of AFFs (see **Fig. 2**). In a study published by Wang and Bhattacharyya[32] in 2011 examining the rates of AFF from 1996 to 2007, the reported age-adjusted rates for subtrochanteric fragility fractures increased among women, from 28.4 in 1999 to 34.2 per 100,000 patient-treatment years in 2007 (an increase of 20.4%), with no significant increase in men. In contrast, typical hip fractures decreased 31.6% (from 1020.5 to 697.4 per 100,000 patient-treatment years) among women and 20.5% (from 424.9 to 337.6 per 100,000 patient-treatment years) among men.

Considerable debate exists regarding the association between AFFs and long-term bisphosphonate use. This debate partly stems from early studies that found a higher risk for femoral shaft fractures in patients with osteoporosis regardless of bisphosphonate treatment,[33–35] suggesting that AFFs are part of the spectrum of fragility (osteoporotic) fractures and that bisphosphonates are not as efficacious in preventing this

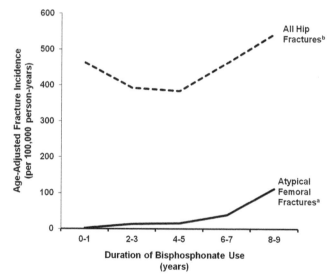

Fig. 2. Age-adjusted incidence of hip fractures and atypical femoral fractures according to duration of bisphosphonate therapy. Data from 1,835,116 patients from a single integrated health care provider. Bisphosphonate exposure was derived from internal pharmacy records. [a] Atypical femoral fractures (continuous line) were identified by diagnostic or procedure codes for the 2007-2011 period and adjudicated by examination of radiographs. [b] Hip fractures (dotted line) were identified by diagnostic codes for the 2007-2009 period and were not further adjudicated. Note the exponential rise in atypical femoral fracture with increasing duration of bisphosphonate therapy. The rate of atypical femoral fractures remains much lower than the rate of hip fractures typically experienced by patients with osteoporosis. (*Adapted from* Dell RM, Adams AL, Greene DF, et al. Incidence of atypical non-traumatic diaphyseal fractures of the femur. J Bone Miner Res 2012 Jul 26. http://dx.doi.org/10.1002/jbmr.1719. [Epub ahead of print]; with permission.)

type of fractures. A major limitation of these early studies is the reliance on International Classification of Diseases (ICD) codes without radiographic adjudication of AFF. Another argument against the theory that AFFs are typical fragility fractures is the recently published finding that the incidence of AFFs (adjudicated by blinded review of radiographs) was independent of bone mineral density and age,[31] unlike the more traditional osteoporotic femoral neck fractures, which are more common in individuals of older age and with lower bone mineral density.

AFFs have also been reported in patients who never used bisphosphonates,[30,31] suggesting that bisphosphonate use is not absolutely necessary for occurrence of these fractures. Nevertheless, the exponential increase in AFF incidence with longer bisphosphonate exposure[31,36,37] and the progressive decline in AFF incidence in individuals who discontinue bisphosphonates[28,37] highly suggest that bisphosphonate use worsens AFF risk. This contention is further supported by the significant increase in AFF incidence in U.S. women since the approval of oral bisphosphonates in 1996, whereas a contemporaneous decline has occurred in the incidence of the more common osteoporotic hip fractures.[29,32] The lack of significant changes in the incidence of AFF and hip fractures in U.S. men during the same period has been attributed to their lower rate of bisphosphonate use.[32]

The pathogenesis of AFF is not entirely understood, but decreased bone turnover has been suggested as the culprit. This notion is interesting when one considers the importance of decreasing bone turnover in the management of patients with osteoporosis, and the fact that not enough evidence shows that suppression is greater in those with than without AFF.[27,38] The process through which decreased bone turnover could lead to increased risk for AFF includes alterations in the normal pattern of collagen cross-linking, microdamage accumulation, increased mineralization, reduced heterogeneity of mineralization, variations in the rate of bone turnover, and reduced vascularity and antiangiogenic effects.[30] A recent publication nicely summarizes these changes and the potential pitfalls associated with the assumption that oversuppression of bone turnover is to be blamed.[39] However, current knowledge regarding AFF suggests that during the process of suppressed bone turnover, increased production of advanced glycation end products may occur, with a reduction in the toughness of bone.[40] Additionally, changes in the normal mineralization pattern to a more homogenous one has been shown in one study,[41] but not in another,[42] to increase the propagation of microcracks. Furthermore, accumulation of bisphosphonates at sites of microdamage could inhibit repair of these microcracks, resulting in their propagation and the development of a stress fracture. Bisphosphonates also seem to inhibit some growth factors that are implicated in angiogenesis,[43] including vascular endothelial growth factor and platelet-derived growth factor, leading to decreased vascularization that could impair fracture healing.

The predisposing risk factors for AFF are not completely understood. Several studies[28,32] have consistently found that long-term bisphosphonate use increases the risk for AFF. Furthermore, the risk conferred by the use of this group of medications seems to be independent of age and bone mineral density.[31] It also seems that after discontinuation of bisphosphonate therapy, a 70% reduction in risk of AFF occurs for every year since the last use.[37] Additional risk factors that have been reported in the literature include Asian ethnicity,[44] the presence of thick cortices before initiation of bisphosphonate therapy,[45] glucocorticoid use,[33] and use of proton pump inhibitors.[46] However, these results are inconsistent, and further evaluation to determine their true contribution to AFF is still needed.

Management of patients with complete AFF includes fracture fixation and initiation of medical management. Optimal surgical management is still unknown, but intramedullary reconstruction with full-length nails is preferred. Medical management should include the discontinuation of bisphosphonates and optimization of calcium and vitamin D intake to around 1000 to 1200 mg/d and at least 800 IU/d, respectively, between diet and supplements. In incomplete AFF, intramedullary nail fixation is recommended in patients with thigh pain, although initiation of teriparatide has been shown in case reports to decrease bone edema and favor the development of cortical bridging.[47–49] Additionally, in 2 patients with delayed healing of incomplete AFF, strontium ranelate led to total closure of the fracture. After an AFF, practitioners must also remain vigilant for the development of symptoms (groin/thigh pain) that suggest an incipient stress fracture in the contralateral limb. Radiographic imaging or MRI of the contralateral femur should be conducted irrespective of the presence of thigh pain.

Osteonecrosis of the Jaw

Osteonecrosis of the jaw (ONJ) was first described in the setting of bisphosphonate use in 2003. Bisphosphonate-associated ONJ was defined by the American Society of Bone and Mineral Research task force in 2007 as exposed bone in the maxillofacial region that does not heal within 8 weeks after identification by a heath care provider in a patient who was receiving or had been exposed to a bisphosphonate and had not had radiation therapy to the craniofacial region.[50] However, ONJ has been described in patients not receiving bisphosphonates, and these patients would not be covered by this definition.

Clinical signs and symptoms of ONJ include pain, swelling, paresthesias, and suppuration, along with soft tissue ulceration and intra- or extraoral sinus tracts. Imaging studies may be normal or show radiolucencies or radio-opacities. The differential diagnosis of bisphosphonate-associated ONJ includes other common intraoral conditions, including periodontal disease, gingivitis or mucositis, temporomandibular joint disease, infectious osteomyelitis, sinusitis, periapical disease caused by a carious infection, osteoradionecrosis, neuralgia-inducing cavitational osteonecrosis, and bone tumors or metastases.

The incidence of ONJ in patients treated with bisphosphonates for osteoporosis remains unknown. During randomized controlled clinical trials, no cases of ONJ were reported. However, several cases of this condition have been reported in the literature in patients receiving bisphosphonates for both benign and malignant conditions. Based on these reports, the American Society for Bone and Mineral Research task force has estimated the incidence of ONJ in patients treated for osteoporosis to be between less than 1 and 10 per 100,000 patient-treatment years.[50] Subsequent studies have reported a similar incidence of 15 to 20 per 100,000 patient-treatment years.[51,52] This finding contrasts with the much higher incidence in patients receiving bisphosphonates for an oncologic indication (1000–10,000 per 100,000 patient-treatment years, depending on the duration of bisphosphonate therapy).

The risk of ONJ in patients treated for a malignancy-related indication is well established, and seems to have a linear relationship with the cumulative dose and/or duration of bisphosphonate therapy.[53] Such a clear relationship has not been well established in patients receiving the lower doses of bisphosphonates currently used for the treatment of osteoporosis. Furthermore, not enough evidence exists to establish a definitive association with the use of bisphosphonates given that ONJ-like lesions occur in patients who have never received bisphosphonates.[54] However, some of the available reports noted a greater risk of ONJ in patients with osteoporosis receiving intravenous bisphosphonates than in those using less-potent oral bisphosphonates.[55] Additionally, suppuration, dental extraction,[50,56] oral bone-manipulating surgery, poor-fitting dental appliances, intraoral trauma, glucocorticoid use, diabetes, preexisting dental or periodontal disease, tobacco/alcohol abuse,[50] and treatment with bisphosphonates for more than 2 years[56] have been identified as potential risk factors.

The pathogenesis of ONJ in patients receiving bisphosphonate therapy remains unclear. Some reports have suggested that ONJ is a result of low bone turnover and microdamage accumulation.[57] Although attractive, this theory has left many unanswered questions, including the fact that well-established ONJ lesions show increased numbers of osteoclasts and that bone lysis is radiographically evident.[58,59] Another alternative explanation has invoked bisphosphonate-induced cellular toxicity leading to impaired epithelial repair on bone surface.[60] In the setting of oral trauma (eg, dental extraction), impaired epithelium provides greater microbial access to the bone surface, increased risk for bone infection, and subsequent biofilm formation. With the development of bone infection, bone resorption, bone necrosis, and exposed bone in the mouth occur, leading to the clinical entity of ONJ.[61]

Treatment of ONJ is entirely empiric and based on available case reports of the condition and on position statements and recommendations made by professional bodies.[50,61–63] Conservative measures, including oral antimicrobial rinses (eg, 0.12% chlorhexidine digluconate), systemic antimicrobial therapy if infection is documented, and pain control, have been advocated.[50] Published case reports also exist of successful therapy with teriparatide[64–66] and hyperbaric oxygen in addition to standard therapy,[67] and of surgical debridement in patients for whom medical management failed,[68] with or without the use of laser.[69] Currently, no published data answer the question of whether stopping bisphosphonates will promote resolution of ONJ. The decision to stop bisphosphonates should therefore be made on an individual basis.

Before initiation of bisphosphonates, patients should be advised to have a dental evaluation, tooth treatment, and full epithelial healing, and undergo treatment of any active oral infections.[63] In patients already receiving bisphosphonates who require dental intervention, the treatment should be conservative, and antibiotic therapy should be considered.[63] Whether bisphosphonates should be stopped is a matter of debate, and currently evidence is insufficient to support discontinuation of therapy. However, practitioners should make decisions on a case-by-case basis.

Upper Gastrointestinal Side Effects

A significant proportion of patients ingesting alendronate in early clinical studies experienced esophageal discomfort and were diagnosed with esophagitis.[70] Endoscopic findings in these patients included chemical esophagitis, erosions or ulcerations, exudative inflammation, and thickening of the esophageal wall, primarily affecting the distal third of the esophagus.[70] Complications included strictures (<1%), and, rarely, hematemesis from esophageal hemorrhage. After early reports of complications, the incidence of esophageal side effects declined significantly once the importance of proper administration was explained to physicians.[71] Subsequently, in the large clinical trials that led to the approval of alendronate for the treatment of postmenopausal osteoporosis, the incidence of upper gastrointestinal tract complaints (especially dyspepsia and abdominal pain) was high but similar in the alendronate and placebo groups (47.5% vs 46.2%; relative risk [RR], 1.02; 95% CI, 0.95–1.10).[72] In these studies, alendronate treatment was not associated with an increased incidence of upper gastrointestinal tract events, even in high-risk subgroups.[72] Esophagitis was more common in patients with preexisting esophageal disorders. In most patients, esophageal complications occur during the first month of oral bisphosphonate therapy, often because the patient takes the medication without an adequate quantity of water or fails to remain upright for 30 or more minutes afterwards. Reducing the frequency of administration (from daily to weekly to monthly dosing) may improve gastrointestinal tolerability, thus reducing the risk of esophageal injury.[73] Switching to an alternate oral or an intravenous bisphosphonate is generally recommended in patients with persistent upper gastrointestinal symptoms.[73]

Esophageal Cancer

Reports of cases of esophageal cancer in patients taking oral bisphosphonates that were voluntarily submitted to the FDA prompted a letter to the editor of the *New England Journal of Medicine* summarizing the available data in 2009.[74] Several oral bisphosphonates were implicated, and pathologic findings included squamous cell carcinoma of the esophagus and adenocarcinoma of the esophagus.[74] The mechanism invoked has implicated a local inflammatory process in response to the response to contact between the esophageal mucosa and oral bisphosphonates, leading to erosive and ulcerative esophagitis and subsequent progression to cancer. These case reports could not prove a causal effect of bisphosphonates in the pathogenesis of esophageal cancer. Subsequently, several reports from the United Kingdom,[75,76] Denmark,[77–79] the United States,[80] and Taiwan[81,82] have evaluated the potential risk of esophageal cancer associated with bisphosphonate use. Most case control studies comparing incidence of esophageal cancer in users versus nonusers of oral bisphosphonates have failed to show a link between bisphosphonate intake and esophageal cancer.[76,77,79,80] Three studies found an increased risk with alendronate use, although the association was not believed to be causal because no dose–response or time relationship was present.[78,81,82] One study comparing previous bisphosphonate use in patients with esophageal cancer and matched controls (without esophageal cancer) found an increased risk when bisphosphonates were prescribed 10 or more times, or for longer than 5 years.[75] Finally, a recently published report found an early decrease in esophageal cancer rates with bisphosphonate use, which may be from greater use of endoscopy before starting alendronate.[79] No excess risk of esophageal cancer death was seen with bisphosphonate use.[79] Overall, problems with surveillance/detection bias, limited information regarding known confounders, and the potential for unmeasured confounding are all limitations of the published epidemiologic studies. Although the FDA acknowledges the conflicting published findings, its most recent communication from July 21, 2011 regarding its "Ongoing Safety Review of Oral Bisphosphonates and Potential Increased Risk of Esophageal Cancer" states that the agency "has not concluded that patients taking oral bisphosphonates have an increased risk of esophageal cancer."[83]

Atrial Fibrillation

Serious atrial fibrillation (Afib) emerged in 2007 as an unexpected but significant side effect of ZA in the phase 3, double-blind, placebo-controlled clinical trial that showed the efficacy of ZA in reducing osteoporotic fractures in postmenopausal women.[8] In this multicenter trial conducted in 3889 women, serious Afib (defined as Afib that either was fatal or led to hospitalization) was reported in 50 women receiving ZA versus 20 women receiving placebo (1.3% vs 0.5%; $P<.001$).[8] These events were uniformly distributed over time, with most occurring more than 30 days after ZA infusion, when blood ZA levels were undetectable. No statistically significant difference in the incidence of stroke, myocardial infarction, or cardiovascular death was noted between the groups. Furthermore, no other electrocardiographic abnormality was noted in the trial, and no plausible mechanism or correlation to electrolyte disturbance was identified. In an extension trial, 1233 postmenopausal women who received ZA for 3 years in that original study were further randomized to 3 additional years of ZA or placebo.[19]

Although numerically more Afib–related serious adverse events were seen in individuals who received a total of 6 years of ZA versus 3 years of ZA followed by 3 years of placebo (2.0% vs 1.1%), this difference was not statistically significant ($P = .26$).[19]

Before publication of the original ZA trial in 2007, there was no signal of cardiac arrhythmias associated with bisphosphonate use, but that publication led to a post hoc review of prior bisphosphonate clinical trials. Reanalysis of the largest placebo-controlled trial with alendronate found no increase in total Afib events ($P = .42$), but noted a trend toward an increase in serious Afib events (47 cases with alendronate vs 31 cases with placebo; hazard ratio [HR], 1.5; 95% CI, 0.97–2.40; $P = .07$).[84] In a recent meta-analysis of all Merck-conducted, placebo-controlled clinical trials of alendronate, no clear association was observed between overall bisphosphonate exposure and the rate of Afib, whether classified as serious (RR, 1.25; 95% CI, 0.82–1.93; $P = .33$) or nonserious (RR, 1.16; 95% CI, 0.87–1.55; $P = .33$).[85] Reanalysis of pooled data from 5 clinical trials of risedronate comprising 15,066 subjects showed no increase in the risk of serious Afib ($P = .49$) or Afib overall ($P = 1$).[86] Likewise, reanalysis of pivotal ibandronate clinical trials involving 8754 patients revealed that the incidence of Afib (ibandronate, 0.8% and placebo, 0.9%) and serious Afib (0.4% for both ibandronate and placebo) was comparable between the ibandronate and placebo groups.[87] One additional placebo-controlled clinical trial with ZA administered after hip fracture also showed no increased risk of overall Afib ($P = .79$) or serious Afib ($P = .84$),[88] and several clinical trials in patients with cancer using ZA at a higher frequency than approved for osteoporosis have not indicated any increased risk of Afib.[89–91] The FDA has reviewed data provided by the manufacturers of the 4 bisphosphonates approved for osteoporosis treatment in the United States regarding 19,687 bisphosphonate-treated patients and 18,358 placebo-treated patients who were followed for 6 months to 3 years. The review found that the occurrence of Afib was rare within each study, and that the absolute difference in event rates between each of the bisphosphonate and placebo arms varied from 0 to 3 per 1000 patient-treatment years.[92]

To overcome the limitations of the placebo-controlled clinical trials that were not designed nor powered to assess rare side effects such as Afib, several observational studies have also examined the association between bisphosphonate use and Afib incidence. A population-based cohort study from Denmark found a significantly higher incidence of serious Afib in fracture patients treated with bisphosphonates compared with matched fracture patients never exposed to bisphosphonates (adjusted HR, 1.13; 95% CI, 1.01–1.26), although the risk among bisphosphonate users was inversely proportional to adherence.[93] In contrast, a separate population-based cohort study from Denmark,[94] and others from the United States,[95] Taiwan,[96] and Korea,[97] have all failed to show an association between bisphosphonate use and incident Afib. One case-control study suggested an increase in Afib risk in U.S. women with past but not current use of alendronate,[98] whereas other studies with a similar case-control design from Denmark[99] or the United Kingdom[100] failed to show such an association. These observational studies vary in terms of which bisphosphonate was studied, method of identifying Afib occurrence, and confounders controlled for, which could explain some of the disparate findings. Furthermore, 4 separately published meta-analyses have pooled results from various studies, again reaching inconsistent conclusions depending on the studies included, with 2 meta-analyses associating bisphosphonate use with an increased incidence of serious Afib,[101,102] and 2 others finding no such association.[103,104]

Several mechanisms have been invoked to explain the potential association between Afib and bisphosphonate use, including the release of inflammatory molecules in the acute phase response after intravenous administration of bisphosph-onates, changes in electrolytes that predispose to arrhythmias (eg, hypocalcemia), and/or atrial structural changes.[105] However, these alternatives remain speculative and none is supported by solid evidence. Currently, the possible association of bisphosphonates with Afib is not well substantiated, and the FDA concluded that "across all studies, no clear association between overall bisphosphonate exposure and the rate of serious or non-serious atrial fibrillation was observed."[92]

Acute Phase Response

Although generally well tolerated, in a significant proportion ($\approx35\%$) of patients the initial doses of intravenous bisphosphonates are associated with a transient acute phase response similar to an influenza-like illness.[8,106] This acute phase response was characterized in placebo-controlled clinical trials by a significantly more common occurrence of fever, chills, diffuse musculoskeletal pain, nausea, fatigue, and head-ache in patients treated with intravenous bisphosphonates than in those treated with placebo.[8,107] Onset of symptoms is approximately 1 day after intravenous infu-sion, with a median duration of approximately 3 days, and symptoms rarely last beyond 2 weeks after infusion.[107] Symptoms are rated as mild or moderate in 90% of cases.[107] Risk factors for acute phase response identified in 1 large multinational study included younger age, non-Japanese Asian ethnicity, and use of nonsteroidal anti-inflammatory drugs, whereas prior exposure to oral bisphosphonate was associ-ated with a lower incidence of acute phase response.[107] Vitamin D insufficiency has also been associated with a higher incidence of acute phase response in adults[108] and children[109] receiving intravenous bisphosphonates. The acute phase response is specific to nitrogen-containing bisphosphonates,[110] and its pathogenesis has been linked to the activation of $\gamma\delta$T lymphocytes, with subsequent release of inter-feron-γ, tumor necrosis factor α, and interleukin-6.[111] Patients with more severe acute phase response exhibited greater rises in these cytokines,[112] strengthening the path-ogenetic link between cytokine release and acute phase response. Although statins prevent bisphosphonate-induced $\gamma\delta$T lymphocyte proliferation and activation in vitro,[113,114] several clinical studies have failed to show a clinical benefit from use of fluvastatin,[115,116] atorvastatin,[117] or rosuvastatin[118] before bisphosphonate infu-sion. In one study, acetaminophen given at 650 mg 4 times daily for 3 days starting before ZA infusion significantly reduced the incidence and severity of post-dose acute phase response, and attenuated increases in serum interleukin-6 and interferon-γ levels at 24 hours compared with placebo and fluvastatin.[115] In view of the self-limited nature of the acute phase response, supportive and symptomatic management with acetaminophen is generally recommended.[119] Although the acute phase response is the most common adverse reaction encountered with intravenous bisphosphonates, it does not seem to impact long-term adherence to bisphospho-nates, because of its mild to moderate severity, short time course, and lower incidence with subsequent treatments.

Ocular Symptoms

Case reports of ocular inflammation occurring in the setting of bisphosphonate use have been reported since the 1990s.[120] Described pathologies range from nonspecific tran-sient conjunctivitis (conjunctival injection) and episcleritis (mild irritation, photophobia, erythema in episcleral vessels) to more serious abnormalities, such as scleritis (severe pain, orbital tenderness, scleral erythema) and anterior uveitis (ocular pain associated with injection of ciliary vessels, photophobia, and blurry vision).[121] Although the exact underlying mechanisms are not entirely understood, bisphosphonate-induced release of inflammatory mediators has been invoked. In some cases, symptoms recur on rechallenge with the same or a different bisphosphonate, corroborating a causal relationship.[120,121]

Ocular symptoms have been described with oral[121–123] and intravenous bisphosphonates,[120,121] and with both nitrogen-containing and non–nitrogen-containing bisphosphonates.[121] In most cases, ocular symptoms occur within 2 to 3 days of exposure to intravenous bisphosphonates[120,121] and 6 to 8 weeks after oral bisphosphonates,[121,122] although reports of onset 1 to 3 years after oral bisphosphonate initiation have been described.[121] Symptoms may be transient, such as in the majority of cases with intravenous bisphosphonates, or persist until discontinuation of oral bisphosphonates. Conjunctivitis might be self-limiting and decrease in intensity over subsequent exposures, providing an option for rechallenge. Potential complications of the more severe presentations (scleritis and anterior uveitis) include development of cataracts, glaucoma, macular edema, and scleral perforation, hence the need for early recognition and appropriate intervention, including bisphosphonate discontinuation.

The incidence of bisphosphonate-associated ocular symptoms has been estimated in 2 large cohort studies. A Canadian cohort examined claims from visits to an ophthalmologist between 2000 and 2007 for 934,147 people, including 10,827 first-time users of bisphosphonates.[122] The incidence rate of uveitis was 29 per 10,000 person-years among first-time bisphosphonate users versus 20 per 10,000 person-years in nonusers. The incidence rates for scleritis were 63 per 10,000 person-years among first-time bisphosphonate users versus 36 per 10,000 person-years in nonusers. Thus, first-time users had a significantly elevated risk of uveitis (adjusted RR of 1.45; 95% CI, 1.25–1.68) and scleritis (adjusted RR, 1.51; 95% CI, 1.34–1.68).[122] A similar RR of 1.23 for scleritis and uveitis was seen among bisphosphonate users in a cohort of U.S. veterans with a 1-year follow-up period.[124]

Severe Musculoskeletal Pain

Between September 1995 (approval of alendronate) and June 2003, 124 cases of severe musculoskeletal pain in the setting of bisphosphonate use were reported to the FDA.[125] Symptoms described included "extreme," "disabling," or "incapacitating" diffuse pain in bones, joints, and/or muscles.[125] These symptoms occurred at different time points after bisphosphonate initiation, and were reported with alendronate use in some cases and risedronate in others, suggesting a class effect.[125] Some patients reported relief of symptoms on bisphosphonate discontinuation, and a subset experienced pain recurrence on rechallenge with the same or a different bisphosphonate, suggesting a causal relationship.[125] These findings prompted the FDA to require that a statement be included on the package insert of all bisphosphonates regarding the possible association of severe musculoskeletal pain, and recommending that patients alert their treating physician if these symptoms occur so that bisphosphonate discontinuation can be considered.[126] Similar, although more transient, musculoskeletal pain has been described as part of the acute phase response ("flu-like symptoms") after intravenous bisphosphonate infusion.

Determinants of the association between bisphosphonate and severe musculoskeletal pain were assessed in a cohort of 26,545 U.S. veterans aged 65 years or older.[127] In this observational study, diffuse musculoskeletal pain identified by ICD-9 code was significantly more common among bisphosphonate users than nonusers (HR, 1.22; 95% CI, 1.04–1.44), but did not lead to more frequent bisphosphonate discontinuation in affected patients.[127] Female sex, depression, anxiety, and the presence of a rheumatic condition were also significantly associated with the development of musculoskeletal pain in this cohort.[127] After adjusting for these and other confounders, bisphosphonate use was no longer significantly associated with the diagnosis of diffuse musculoskeletal pain in multivariate analysis (HR, 1.10; 95% CI, 0.93–1.30).[127] Similarly, in placebo-controlled clinical trials with oral bisphosphonates, the incidence of severe musculoskeletal pain was not different in the bisphosphonate versus placebo groups. Taken together, these findings do not suggest a strong association between bisphosphonate use and severe musculoskeletal pain, and no plausible mechanisms have been proven to explain such an association. Nevertheless, in patients who develop severe musculoskeletal pain with bisphosphonate use, discontinuation should be considered.

Renal Insufficiency

Administration of bisphosphonates in high doses and at a rapid rate in animal models induces a variety of adverse renal effects, from glomerular sclerosis to acute tubular necrosis.[128] In humans, the most common adverse renal effect is a transient rise in serum creatinine with a subsequent return to baseline. This complication seems to be related to the maximum bisphosphonate plasma concentration (C_{max}), because rapid infusion (5 minutes) of monthly pamidronate or ZA in oncology trials induced acute rises in serum creatinine, which was not seen with slower infusion rates (15 or 30 minutes) of the same doses.[129,130] Pathologic findings in the limited cases in which a kidney biopsy was obtained include loss of tubular cell polarization, loss of brush border and apoptosis of proximal tubular cells, and increased proliferation, all hallmarks of acute tubular necrosis.[131] At the dose and infusion rate approved for the treatment of osteoporosis (5 mg infused 15 minutes once a year), intravenous ZA induced transient increases in serum creatinine in a small but significant number of subjects, with return of serum creatinine to baseline levels before the next annual infusion.[8] The incidence of renal adverse events was similarly low in the Dosing Intravenous Administration trial of intravenous ibandronate.[106] After postmarketing reports of acute renal failure in patients with osteoporosis treated with intravenous ZA, the FDA sent a newsletter to physicians in 2011 reminding them of this potential risk.[132] The FDA also requested a label revision, stating that Reclast is contraindicated in patients with creatinine clearance less than 35 mL/min or those with evidence of acute renal impairment. Screening of patients before administering Reclast to identify those at risk (use of diuretics or nephrotoxic drugs at the same time as Reclast, or severe dehydration occurring before or after Reclast is given) was also recommended. Still, the overall risk of kidney damage in patients receiving intravenous bisphosphonates for osteoporosis is very small, and can be further reduced through ensuring adequate hydration and use of appropriate infusion times.[133,134] Glomerulosclerosis with nephrotic range proteinuria has been described in very few cases of patients receiving intravenous pamidronate,[131,135,136] oral alendronate,[137] and ZA.[138] This renal complication of bisphosphonates is extremely rare and was not noted during any of the pivotal clinical trials.

Hypocalcemia

With the widespread use of bisphosphonates for various conditions and the introduction of more potent compounds, symptomatic hypocalcemia has been recognized as a complication associated with their use.[139] Despite patients with diseases affecting bone metabolism being excluded from clinical trials of oral alendronate[140,141] and risedronate,[142] and the provision of calcium supplements to all participants in these trials, mild, transient, but statistically significant declines in serum calcium were noted with bisphosphonate use. In clinical trials of intravenously administered bisphosphonates, mild asymptomatic hypocalcemia was noted in 0.2% of patients with osteoporosis.[143] In patients with cancer, Chennuru and colleagues[144] reported the occurrence of hypocalcemia after 10% of 546 ZA infusions, with symptomatic hypocalcaemia requiring intravenous calcium supplementation in 8% of patients, despite ZA dose adjustment for creatinine clearance and prophylactic administration of oral calcium and vitamin D. Bisphosphonate-induced severe hypocalcemia has also been associated with the occurrence of seizures in several cases, likely through lowering the seizure threshold in patients with known epilepsy.[145]

Mechanistically, bisphosphonates reduce calcium efflux from bone through inhibiting osteoclastic bone resorption, which is normally followed by a compensatory increase in parathyroid hormone secretion.[146] This process in turn enhances the distal renal tubular calcium reabsorption and stimulates intestinal calcium absorption through increased renal production of 1,25-dihydroxyvitamin D.[146] Hypocalcemia after bisphosphonate exposure has been associated with conditions that impair these compensatory mechanisms (eg, hypoparathyroidism and/or vitamin D deficiency) and with reduced renal function (which lowers bisphosphonate clearance, resulting in potentially greater antiresorptive action).[139]

Case reports and series have reported vitamin D deficiency and/or hypoparathyroidism to be risk factors for bisphosphonate-induced hypocalcemia.[139] In one study, more patients who became hypocalcemic developed worsening creatinine clearance post-ZA, suggesting that renal impairment occurring in the days after administration may increase the risk of hypocalcemia.[144] Hypocalcemia tends to develop earlier with the use of more potent bisphosphonates.[139] Hypomagnesemia occurs frequently in patients with bisphosphonate-induced hypocalcemia,[144] and may contribute to this complication through blunting the compensatory increase in parathyroid hormone secretion. The product labels for approved bisphosphonates include specific warnings against their use in patients with these risk factors. Assessing renal function and vitamin D stores before bisphosphonate initiation has been suggested in patients for whom this therapy is contemplated, partly to prevent hypocalcemia.

OVERALL EFFICACY VERSUS SAFETY CONSIDERATION

Recent concerns over the potential side effects of bisphosphonate use (**Table 2**) along with the available data regarding the long-term efficacy of these medications have led to recent reconsideration of the optimal treatment duration with these agents. In placebo-controlled clinical trials lasting 3 to 4 years, bisphosphonates have been shown to significantly reduce osteoporotic fractures. The absolute fracture reduction with bisphosphonates depends on the baseline risk and site of fracture (vertebral vs nonvertebral) (**Fig. 3**, left panel).[6,21,147] In this time frame of 3 to 4 years, the benefits of bisphosphonates clearly outweigh the risks (see **Fig. 3**, right panel). At the same time, very limited data exist on the antifracture efficacy beyond 5 years of therapy, except in high-risk patients (defined as those with prior osteoporotic fracture or persistently low femoral neck T-score). In other patients, a "drug holiday" or "bisphosphonate holiday" (ie, a period during which bisphosphonate intake is suspended) has been suggested,[148] and more recently endorsed in guidelines from the American Association of Clinical Endocrinologists.[149] Advocates of a drug holiday have argued that the efficacy of bisphosphonates has not been shown beyond 5 years of therapy for most low-risk patients, and that the incidence of side effects such as AFF and ONJ increases with prolonged bisphosphonate use. Opponents of the drug holiday concept argue that no data show loss of efficacy with prolonged use, and that the risk of complications (AFF and ONJ) is very small compared with the incidence of

Table 2
Overview of side effects associated with bisphosphonates

Side Effect	Upper Gastrointestinal Tract Discomfort	Acute Phase Response	Renal Insufficiency	AFFs	Osteonecrosis of the Jaw	Ocular Inflammation	Severe Musculoskeletal Pain	Esophageal Cancer	Afib
Incidence	Common with oral BPs	Common with initial IV BP infusion	Rare, mostly with IV BPs	Rare[a]	Rare[a]	Rare[a]	Rare[a]	Rare[a]	Rare, only seen in one controlled study with ZA
Strength of association	Definite	Definite	Probable	Probable	Probable	Probable	Possible[b]	Questionable[c]	Questionable[d]
Mechanism	Irritation of upper gastrointestinal mucosa	Activation of γδT lymphocytes	FSGS with nephrotic syndrome, other ? mechanisms	Unknown at risk ? patients changes ? in bone material properties	Unknown impaired ? repair against oral infections impaired ? mucosal healing	Release of inflammatory mediators	Unknown	Esophageal inflammation with oral BPs	Unknown inflammation ? changes in electrolytes or in heart structure
Comments	Increased incidence of nausea, dyspepsia, abdominal pain, and acid regurgitation	Incidence decreases with repeated dosing	FSGS case reports with oral and IV BP, Higher risk of rise in SCr in IV BP trials	Incidence increases with prolonged BP use, decreases with BP cessation	Incidence increases with prolonged BP use	Scleritis, uveitis, conjunctivitis, other symptoms Cases of recurrence on rechallenge with same or different BP	Severe bone, joint, muscle pain Variable time to onset after starting BP Subset with pain recurrence on BP rechallenge	Oral BP users at higher risk for upper gastrointestinal symptoms and thus for undergoing endoscopy ? detection bias	Signficantly increased risk seen in a single randomized placebo-controlled trial. Data from observational studies are conflicting.

Abbreviations: BP, bisphosphonate; FSGS, focal segmental glomerular sclerosis; IV, intravenous; SCr, serum creatinine; ZA, zoledronic acid.

[a] No difference in incidence compared with placebo in clinical trials lasting 3 to 5 years.

[b] No difference in incidence of severe musculoskeletal pain between bisphosphonate versus placebo groups in clinical trials. No association with bisphosphonate use after adjusting for potential confounders in one large observational study. Some patients report relief of symptoms on bisphosphonate discontinuation and a subset report pain recurrence on rechallenge with the same or a different bisphosphonate.

[c] Most studies have either shown no significant association with bisphosphonate use, or no dose and duration relationship with bisphosphonate use.

[d] Most clinical trials and observational studies have shown no significant association between bisphosphonate use and Afib.

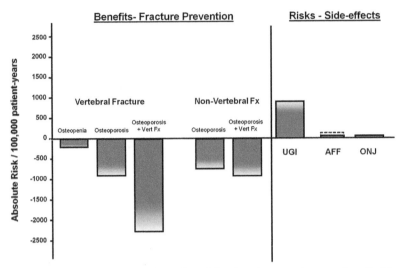

Fig. 3. Comparison of risks versus benefits of bisphosphonate therapy. Benefit (fracture reduction) with bisphosphonate therapy depends on baseline risk of fracture (lowest risk in patients with osteopenia, highest risk in patients with osteoporosis and prevalent vertebral fracture, intermediate risk in osteoporotic patients with no prevalent vertebral fracture) and site of fracture (radiographic vertebral fracture vs nonvertebral fracture). Data based on 3- and 4-year placebo-controlled clinical trials of alendronate therapy. Incidence of side effects of bisphosphonates, including upper gastrointestinal tract symptoms, ONJ, and AFF. Incidence of AFF after 3 years of bisphosphonate therapy is shown in the gray bar, whereas its higher incidence after 10 years of therapy is indicated by the dotted lines. (*Data from* Quandt SA, Thompson DE, Schneider DL, et al. Effect of alendronate on vertebral fracture risk in women with bone mineral density T scores of -1.6 to -2.5 at the femoral neck: the Fracture Intervention Trial. Mayo Clin Proc 2005;80:343–9; Black DM, Cummings SR, Karpf DB, et al. Randomised trial of effect of alendronate on risk of fracture in women with existing vertebral fractures. Fracture Intervention Trial Research Group. Lancet 1996;348:1535–41; Liberman UA, Weiss SR, Broll J, et al. Effect of oral alendronate on bone mineral density and the incidence of fractures in postmenopausal osteoporosis. The Alendronate Phase III Osteoporosis Treatment Study Group. N Engl J Med 1995;333:1437–43; and Dell RM, Adams AL, Greene DF, et al. Incidence of atypical nontraumatic diaphyseal fractures of the femur. J Bone Miner Res 2012, in press.)

osteoporotic fractures that can be prevented with bisphosphonate use. At an FDA advisory committee hearing held in September 2011,[1] no consensus regarding optimal duration of bisphosphonate therapy was reached. Still, the product labels of currently approved bisphosphonates contain the following "Important Limitation of Use" statement: "The optimal duration of use has not been determined. All patients on bisphosphonate therapy should have the need for continued therapy reevaluated on a periodic basis." The authors agree with the need for periodic reevaluation of the need for continued bisphosphonate therapy beyond 5 years. Considerations in this decision should include the patient's risk of fracture, response to therapy, comorbidities, and preferences.

Many unanswered questions remain regarding the optimal duration of initial bisphosphonate therapy, its safety and efficacy in long-term users, and the optimal duration of a bisphosphonate holiday and its impact on fracture risk and potential reduction of side effects, such as AFF and ONJ. Given the differences in pharmacologic properties of the various bisphosphonates, drug-specific rather than class-specific recommendations may be needed. More research is also needed to address the potential mechanisms through which ONJ and AFF occur, which may lead to preventative measures or optimal treatment strategies. Finally, whether a causal association exists between bisphosphonates and esophageal cancer and Afib must be determined.

SUMMARY

Bisphosphonates remain a cornerstone for fracture reduction in patients with osteoporosis. Potentially serious side effects have been linked to bisphosphonate use, including ONJ and AFF. The risk of ONJ in patients with osteoporosis ranges between 0.6 and 20 per 100,000 patient-treatment years, whereas the risk of atypical subtrochanteric fractures is between 2 and 120 per 100,000 patient-treatment years and increases with duration of bisphosphonate therapy. Bisphosphonates are unlikely to increase the risk of Afib or esophageal cancer based on the currently available data. Overall, bisphosphonate-associated risks are significantly lower than the incidence of hip fracture from untreated osteoporosis. Based on the current understanding of bisphosphonate-associated side effects and the significant benefits from bisphosphonate therapy, both in primary and secondary prevention of fractures, one should continue to treat patients with osteoporosis using bisphosphonates, while remaining cautious and reassessing the need for continued bisphosphonate therapy beyond 3 to 5 years on an annual basis.

REFERENCES

1. Background document for meeting of Advisory Committee for Reproductive Health Drugs and Drug Safety and Risk Management Advisory Committee. Available at: http://www.fda.gov/downloads/AdvisoryCommittees/CommitteesMeetingMaterials/Drugs/DrugSafetyandRiskManagementAdvisoryCommittee/UCM270958.pdf. Accessed September 17, 2012.
2. Rodan GA, Fleisch HA. Bisphosphonates: mechanisms of action. J Clin Invest 1996;97:2692-6.
3. Sato M, Grasser W, Endo N, et al. Bisphosphonate action. Alendronate localization in rat bone and effects on osteoclast ultrastructure. J Clin Invest 1991;88:2095-105.
4. Khan SA, Kanis JA, Vasikaran S, et al. Elimination and biochemical responses to intravenous alendronate in postmenopausal osteoporosis. J Bone Miner Res 1997;12:1700-7.
5. Russell RG, Watts NB, Ebetino FH, et al. Mechanisms of action of bisphosphonates: similarities and differences and their potential influence on clinical efficacy. Osteoporos Int 2008;19:733-59.
6. Black DM, Cummings SR, Karpf DB, et al. Randomised trial of effect of alendronate on risk of fracture in women with existing vertebral fractures. Fracture Intervention Trial Research Group. Lancet 1996;348:1535-41.
7. Reginster J, Minne HW, Sorensen OH, et al. Randomized trial of the effects of risedronate on vertebral fractures in women with established postmenopausal osteoporosis. Vertebral Efficacy with Risedronate Therapy (VERT) Study Group. Osteoporos Int 2000;11:83-91.
8. Black DM, Delmas PD, Eastell R, et al. Once-yearly zoledronic acid for treatment of postmenopausal osteoporosis. N Engl J Med 2007;356:1809-22.

9. Chesnut IC, Skag A, Christiansen C, et al. Effects of oral ibandronate administered daily or intermittently on fracture risk in postmenopausal osteoporosis. J Bone Miner Res 2004;19:1241–9.

10. Harris ST, Watts NB, Genant HK, et al. Effects of risedronate treatment on vertebral and nonvertebral fractures in women with postmenopausal osteoporosis: a randomized controlled trial. Vertebral Efficacy with Risedronate Therapy (VERT) Study Group. JAMA 1999;282:1344–52.

11. McClung MR, Geusens P, Miller PD, et al. Effect of risedronate on the risk of hip fracture in elderly women. Hip Intervention Program Study Group. N Engl J Med 2001;344:333–40.

12. Harris ST, Blumentals WA, Miller PD. Ibandronate and the risk of non-vertebral and clinical fractures in women with postmenopausal osteoporosis: results of a meta-analysis of phase III studies. Curr Med Res Opin 2008;24:237–45.

13. Silverman SL, Watts NB, Delmas PD, et al. Effectiveness of bisphosphonates on nonvertebral and hip fractures in the first year of therapy: the risedronate and alendronate (REAL) cohort study. Osteoporos Int 2007;18:25–34.

14. Silverman SL. Osteoporosis therapies: evidence from health-care databases and observational population studies. Calcif Tissue Int 2010;87:375–84.

15. Miller PD. Bone density and markers of bone turnover in predicting fracture risk and how changes in these measures predict fracture risk reduction. Curr Osteoporos Rep 2005;3:103–10.

16. Watts NB, Lewiecki EM, Bonnick SL, et al. Clinical value of monitoring BMD in patients treated with bisphosphonates for osteoporosis. J Bone Miner Res 2009;24:1643–6.

17. Black DM, Schwartz AV, Ensrud KE, et al. Effects of continuing or stopping alendronate after 5 years of treatment: the Fracture Intervention Trial Long-term Extension (FLEX): a randomized trial. JAMA 2006;296:2927–38.

18. Schwartz AV, Bauer DC, Cummings SR, et al. Efficacy of continued alendronate for fractures in women with and without prevalent vertebral fracture: the FLEX trial. J Bone Miner Res 2010;25:976–82.

19. Black DM, Reid IR, Boonen S, et al. The effect of 3 versus 6 years of zoledronic acid treatment of osteoporosis: a randomized extension to the HORIZON-Pivotal Fracture Trial (PFT). J Bone Miner Res 2012;27:243–54.

20. Eastell R, Hannon RA, Wenderoth D, et al. Effect of stopping risedronate after long-term treatment on bone turnover. J Clin Endocrinol Metab 2011;96:3367–73.

21. Liberman UA, Weiss SR, Broll J, et al. Effect of oral alendronate on bone mineral density and the incidence of fractures in postmenopausal osteoporosis. The Alendronate Phase III Osteoporosis Treatment Study Group. N Engl J Med 1995;333:1437–43.

22. Ravn P, Clemmesen B, Riis BJ, et al. The effect on bone mass and bone markers of different doses of ibandronate: a new bisphosphonate for prevention and treatment of postmenopausal osteoporosis: a 1-year, randomized, double-blind, placebo-controlled dose-finding study. Bone 1996;19:527–33.

23. Reid IR, Brown JP, Burckhardt P, et al. Intravenous zoledronic acid in postmenopausal women with low bone mineral density. N Engl J Med 2002;346:653–61.

24. Odvina CV, Zerwekh JE, Rao DS, et al. Severely suppressed bone turnover: a potential complication of alendronate therapy. J Clin Endocrinol Metab 2005;90:1294–301.

25. Donnelly E, Meredith DS, Nguyen JT, et al. Reduced cortical bone compositional heterogeneity with bisphosphonate treatment in postmenopausal women with

intertrochanteric and subtrochanteric fractures. J Bone Miner Res 2012;27: 672–8.

26. Goh SK, Yang KY, Koh JS, et al. Subtrochanteric insufficiency fractures in patients on alendronate therapy: a caution. J Bone Joint Surg Br 2007;89: 349–53.

27. Armamento-Villareal R, Napoli N, Diemer K, et al. Bone turnover in bone biopsies of patients with low-energy cortical fractures receiving bisphosphonates: a case series. Calcif Tissue Int 2009;85:37–44.

28. Park-Wyllie LY, Mamdani MM, Juurlink DN, et al. Bisphosphonate use and the risk of subtrochanteric or femoral shaft fractures in older women. JAMA 2011; 305:783–9.

29. Feldstein AC, Black D, Perrin N, et al. Incidence and demography of femur fractures with and without atypical features. J Bone Miner Res 2012;27:977–86.

30. Shane E, Burr D, Ebeling PR, et al. Atypical subtrochanteric and diaphyseal femoral fractures: report of a task force of the American Society for Bone and Mineral Research. J Bone Miner Res 2010;25:2267–94.

31. Dell RM, Adams AL, Greene DF, et-al. Incidence of atypical nontraumatic diaphyseal fractures of the femur. J Bone Miner Res, in press. doi:http://dx.doi.org/10.1002/jbmr.1719.

32. Wang Z, Bhattacharyya T. Trends in incidence of subtrochanteric fragility fractures and bisphosphonate use among the US elderly, 1996-2007. J Bone Miner Res 2011;26:553–60.

33. Abrahamsen B, Eiken P, Eastell R. Subtrochanteric and diaphyseal femur fractures in patients treated with alendronate: a register-based national cohort study. J Bone Miner Res 2009;24:1095–102.

34. Vestergaard P, Schwartz F, Rejnmark L, et al. Risk of femoral shaft and subtrochanteric fractures among users of bisphosphonates and raloxifene. Osteoporos Int 2011;22:993–1001.

35. Nieves JW, Bilezikian JP, Lane JM, et al. Fragility fractures of the hip and femur: incidence and patient characteristics. Osteoporos Int 2010;21:399–408.

36. Meier RP, Perneger TV, Stern R, et al. Increasing occurrence of atypical femoral fractures associated with bisphosphonate use atypical femoral fractures and bisphosphonate use. Arch Intern Med 2012;172:930–6.

37. Schilcher J, Michaelsson K, Aspenberg P. Bisphosphonate use and atypical fractures of the femoral shaft. N Engl J Med 2011;364:1728–37.

38. Ing-Lorenzini K, Desmeules J, Plachta O, et al. Low-energy femoral fractures associated with the long-term use of bisphosphonates: a case series from a Swiss university hospital. Drug Saf 2009;32:775–85.

39. Compston J. Pathophysiology of atypical femoral fractures and osteonecrosis of the jaw. Osteoporos Int 2011;22:2951–61.

40. Allen MR, Gineyts E, Leeming DJ, et al. Bisphosphonates alter trabecular bone collagen cross-linking and isomerization in beagle dog vertebra. Osteoporos Int 2008;19:329–37.

41. Donnelly E, Meredith DS, Nguyen JT, et al. Reduced cortical bone compositional heterogeneity with bisphosphonate treatment in postmenopausal women with intertrochanteric and subtrochanteric fractures. J Bone Miner Res 2012;27: 672–8.

42. Somford MP, Draijer FW, Thomassen BJ, et al. Bilateral fractures of the femur diaphysis in a patient with rheumatoid arthritis on long-term treatment with alendronate: clues to the mechanism of increased bone fragility. J Bone Miner Res 2009;24:1736–40.

43. Fournier P, Boissier S, Filleur S, et al. Bisphosphonates inhibit angiogenesis in vitro and testosterone-stimulated vascular regrowth in the ventral prostate in castrated rats. Cancer Res 2002;62:6538–44.
44. Lo JC, Huang SY, Lee GA, et al. Clinical correlates of atypical femoral fracture. Bone 2012;51:181–4.
45. Kwek EB, Goh SK, Koh JS, et al. An emerging pattern of subtrochanteric stress fractures: a long-term complication of alendronate therapy? Injury 2008;39:224–31.
46. Fournier MR, Targownik LE, Leslie WD. Proton pump inhibitors, osteoporosis, and osteoporosis-related fractures. Maturitas 2009;64:9–13.
47. Gomberg SJ, Wustrack RL, Napoli N, et al. Teriparatide, vitamin D, and calcium healed bilateral subtrochanteric stress fractures in a postmenopausal woman with a 13-year history of continuous alendronate therapy. J Clin Endocrinol Metab 2011;96:1627–32.
48. Donnelly E, Saleh A, Unnanuntana A, et al. Atypical femoral fractures: epidemiology, etiology, and patient management. Curr Opin Support Palliat Care 2012; 6:348–54.
49. Carvalho NN, Voss LA, Almeida MO, et al. Atypical femoral fractures during prolonged use of bisphosphonates: short-term responses to strontium ranelate and teriparatide. J Clin Endocrinol Metab 2011;96:2675–80.
50. Khosla S, Burr D, Cauley J, et al. Bisphosphonate-associated osteonecrosis of the jaw: report of a task force of the American Society for Bone and Mineral Research. J Bone Miner Res 2007;22:1479–91.
51. Solomon DH, Mercer E, Woo SB, et-al. Defining the epidemiology of bisphosphonate-associated osteonecrosis of the jaw: prior work and current challenges. Osteoporos Int, in press.
52. Tennis P, Rothman KJ, Bohn RL, et al. Incidence of osteonecrosis of the jaw among users of bisphosphonates with selected cancers or osteoporosis. Pharmacoepidemiol Drug Saf 2012;21:810–7.
53. Durie BG, Katz M, Crowley J. Osteonecrosis of the jaw and bisphosphonates. N Engl J Med 2005;353:99–102 [discussion: 99].
54. Fellows JL, Rindal DB, Barasch A, et al. ONJ in two dental practice-based research network regions. J Dent Res 2011;90:433–8.
55. Woo SB, Hellstein JW, Kalmar JR. Narrative [corrected] review: bisphosphonates and osteonecrosis of the jaws. Ann Intern Med 2006;144:753–61.
56. Barasch A, Cunha-Cruz J, Curro FA, et al. Risk factors for osteonecrosis of the jaws: a case-control study from the CONDOR dental PBRN. J Dent Res 2011;90: 439–44.
57. Kyrgidis A, Verrou E. Fatigue in bone: a novel phenomenon attributable to bisphosphonate use. Bone 2010;46:556 [author reply: 7–8].
58. Dodson TB, Raje NS, Caruso PA, et al. Case records of the Massachusetts General Hospital. Case 9-2008. A 65-year-old woman with a nonhealing ulcer of the jaw. N Engl J Med 2008;358:1283–91.
59. Krishnan A, Arslanoglu A, Yildirm N, et al. Imaging findings of bisphosphonate-related osteonecrosis of the jaw with emphasis on early magnetic resonance imaging findings. J Comput Assist Tomogr 2009;33:298–304.
60. Reid IR, Bolland MJ, Grey AB. Is bisphosphonate-associated osteonecrosis of the jaw caused by soft tissue toxicity? Bone 2007;41:318–20.
61. Dental management of patients receiving oral bisphosphonate therapy: expert panel recommendations. J Am Dent Assoc 2006;137:1144–50.
62. American College of Rheumatology, editor. Bisphosphonate-associated osteonecrosis of the jaw. Atlanta (GA): American College of Rheumatology; 2006.

63. Rizzoli R, Burlet N, Cahall D, et al. Osteonecrosis of the jaw and bisphosphonate treatment for osteoporosis. Bone 2008;42:841-7.

64. Iwamoto J, Yago K, Sato Y, et al. Teriparatide therapy for bisphosphonate-associated osteonecrosis of the jaw in an elderly Japanese woman with severe osteoporosis. Clin Drug Investig 2012;32:547-53.

65. Lau AN, Adachi JD. Resolution of osteonecrosis of the jaw after teriparatide [recombinant human PTH-(1-34)] therapy. J Rheumatol 2009;36:1835-7.

66. Cheung A, Seeman E. Teriparatide therapy for alendronate-associated osteonecrosis of the jaw. N Engl J Med 2010;363:2473-4.

67. Freiberger JJ, Padilla-Burgos R, McGraw T, et al. What is the role of hyperbaric oxygen in the management of bisphosphonate-related osteonecrosis of the jaw: a randomized controlled trial of hyperbaric oxygen as an adjunct to surgery and antibiotics. J Oral Maxillofac Surg 2012;70:1573-83.

68. Voss PJ, Joshi Oshero J, Kovalova-Muller A, et-al. Surgical treatment of bisphosphonate-associated osteonecrosis of the jaw: technical report and follow up of 21 patients. J Craniomaxillofac Surg, in press.

69. Vescovi P, Merigo E, Meleti M, et al. Bisphosphonates-related osteonecrosis of the jaws: a concise review of the literature and a report of a single-centre experience with 151 patients. J Oral Pathol Med 2012;41:214-21.

70. de Groen PC, Lubbe DF, Hirsch LJ, et al. Esophagitis associated with the use of alendronate. N Engl J Med 1996;335:1016-21.

71. Cryer B, Bauer DC. Oral bisphosphonates and upper gastrointestinal tract problems: what is the evidence? Mayo Clin Proc 2002;77:1031-43.

72. Bauer DC, Black D, Ensrud K, et al. Upper gastrointestinal tract safety profile of alendronate: the fracture intervention trial. Arch Intern Med 2000;160:517-25.

73. Strampel W, Emkey R, Civitelli R. Safety considerations with bisphosphonates for the treatment of osteoporosis. Drug Saf 2007;30:755-63.

74. Wysowski DK. Reports of esophageal cancer with oral bisphosphonate use. N Engl J Med 2009;360:89-90.

75. Green J, Czanner G, Reeves G, et al. Oral bisphosphonates and risk of cancer of oesophagus, stomach, and colorectum: case-control analysis within a UK primary care cohort. BMJ 2010;341:c4444.

76. Cardwell CR, Abnet CC, Cantwell MM, et al. Exposure to oral bisphosphonates and risk of esophageal cancer. JAMA 2010;304:657-63.

77. Abrahamsen B, Eiken P, Eastell R. More on reports of esophageal cancer with oral bisphosphonate use. N Engl J Med 2009;360:1789 [author reply: 91-2].

78. Vestergaard P. Occurrence of gastrointestinal cancer in users of bisphosphonates and other antiresorptive drugs against osteoporosis. Calcif Tissue Int 2011;89:434-41.

79. Abrahamsen B, Pazianas M, Eiken P, et al. Esophageal and gastric cancer incidence and mortality in alendronate users. J Bone Miner Res 2012;27:679-86.

80. Solomon DH, Patrick A, Brookhart MA. More on reports of esophageal cancer with oral bisphosphonate use. N Engl J Med 2009;360:1789-90 [author reply: 91-2].

81. Chen YM, Chen DY, Chen LK, et al. Alendronate and risk of esophageal cancer: a nationwide population-based study in Taiwan. J Am Geriatr Soc 2011;59: 2379-81.

82. Ho YF, Lin JT, Wu CY. Oral bisphosphonates and risk of esophageal cancer: a dose-intensity analysis in a nationwide population. Cancer Epidemiol Biomarkers Prev 2012;21:993-5.

83. U.S. Food and Drug Administration. FDA Drug Safety Communication: Ongoing safety review of oral osteoporosis drugs (bisphosphonates) and potential

increased risk of esophageal cancer. Available at: http://www.fda.gov/drugs/drugsafety/ucm263320.htm. Accessed September 17, 2012.

84. Cummings SR, Schwartz AV, Black DM. Alendronate and atrial fibrillation. N Engl J Med 2007;356:1895–6.

85. Barrett-Connor E, Swern AS, Hustad CM, et al. Alendronate and atrial fibrillation: a meta-analysis of randomized placebo-controlled clinical trials. Osteoporos Int 2012;23:233–45.

86. Karam R, Camm J, McClung M. Yearly zoledronic acid in postmenopausal osteoporosis. N Engl J Med 2007;357:712–3 [author reply: 4–5].

87. Lewiecki EM, Cooper C, Thompson E, et al. Ibandronate does not increase risk of atrial fibrillation in analysis of pivotal clinical trials. Int J Clin Pract 2010;64: 821–6.

88. Lyles KW, Colon-Emeric CS, Magaziner JS, et al. Zoledronic acid and clinical fractures and mortality after hip fracture. N Engl J Med 2007;357: 1799–809.

89. Bundred NJ, Campbell ID, Davidson N, et al. Effective inhibition of aromatase inhibitor-associated bone loss by zoledronic acid in postmenopausal women with early breast cancer receiving adjuvant letrozole: ZO-FAST Study results. Cancer 2008;112:1001–10.

90. Hershman DL, McMahon DJ, Crew KD, et al. Zoledronic acid prevents bone loss in premenopausal women undergoing adjuvant chemotherapy for early-stage breast cancer. J Clin Oncol 2008;26:4739–45.

91. Smith MR, Eastham J, Gleason DM, et al. Randomized controlled trial of zoledronic acid to prevent bone loss in men receiving androgen deprivation therapy for nonmetastatic prostate cancer. J Urol 2003;169:2008–12.

92. U.S. Food and Drug Administration. Update of safety review follow-up to the October 1, 2007 early communication about the ongoing safety review of bisphosphonates. Available at: http://www.fda.gov/Drugs/DrugSafety/PostmarketDrugSafetyInformationforPatientsandProviders/DrugSafetyInformationforHeathcareProfessionals/ucm136201.htm. Accessed September 17, 2012.

93. Abrahamsen B, Eiken P, Brixen K. Atrial fibrillation in fracture patients treated with oral bisphosphonates. J Intern Med 2009;265:581–92.

94. Vestergaard P, Schwartz K, Pinholt EM, et al. Risk of atrial fibrillation associated with use of bisphosphonates and other drugs against osteoporosis: a cohort study. Calcif Tissue Int 2010;86:335–42.

95. Bunch TJ, Anderson JL, May HT, et al. Relation of bisphosphonate therapies and risk of developing atrial fibrillation. Am J Cardiol 2009;103:824–8.

96. Huang WF, Tsai YW, Wen YW, et al. Osteoporosis treatment and atrial fibrillation: alendronate versus raloxifene. Menopause 2010;17:57–63.

97. Rhee CW, Lee J, Oh S, et al. Use of bisphosphonate and risk of atrial fibrillation in older women with osteoporosis. Osteoporos Int 2012;23:247–54.

98. Heckbert SR, Li G, Cummings SR, et al. Use of alendronate and risk of incident atrial fibrillation in women. Arch Intern Med 2008;168:826–31.

99. Sorensen HT, Christensen S, Mehnert F, et al. Use of bisphosphonates among women and risk of atrial fibrillation and flutter: population based case-control study. BMJ 2008;336:813–6.

100. Grosso A, Douglas I, Hingorani A, et al. Oral bisphosphonates and risk of atrial fibrillation and flutter in women: a self-controlled case-series safety analysis. PLoS One 2009;4:e4720.

101. Loke YK, Jeevanantham V, Singh S. Bisphosphonates and atrial fibrillation: systematic review and meta-analysis. Drug Saf 2009;32:219–28.

102. Bhuriya R, Singh M, Molnar J, et al. Bisphosphonate use in women and the risk of atrial fibrillation: a systematic review and meta-analysis. Int J Cardiol 2010; 142:213–7.
103. Mak A, Cheung MW, Ho RC, et al. Bisphosphonates and atrial fibrillation: bayesian meta-analyses of randomized controlled trials and observational studies. BMC Musculoskelet Disord 2009;10:113.
104. Kim SY, Kim MJ, Cadarette SM, et al. Bisphosphonates and risk of atrial fibrillation: a meta-analysis. Arthritis Res Ther 2010;12:R30.
105. Howard PA, Barnes BJ, Vacek JL, et al. Impact of bisphosphonates on the risk of atrial fibrillation. Am J Cardiovasc Drugs 2010;10:359–67.
106. Delmas PD, Adami S, Strugala C, et al. Intravenous ibandronate injections in postmenopausal women with osteoporosis: one-year results from the dosing intravenous administration study. Arthritis Rheum 2006;54:1838–46.
107. Reid IR, Gamble GD, Mesenbrink P, et al. Characterization of and risk factors for the acute-phase response after zoledronic acid. J Clin Endocrinol Metab 2010; 95:4380–7.
108. Bertoldo F, Pancheri S, Zenari S, et al. Serum 25-hydroxyvitamin D levels modulate the acute-phase response associated with the first nitrogen-containing bisphosphonate infusion. J Bone Miner Res 2010;25:447–54.
109. Srivastava T, Dai H, Haney CJ, et al. Serum 25-hydroxyvitamin D level and acute-phase reaction following initial intravenous bisphosphonate. J Bone Miner Res 2011;26:437–8.
110. Olson K, Van Poznak C. Significance and impact of bisphosphonate-induced acute phase responses. J Oncol Pharm Pract 2007;13:223–9.
111. Thompson K, Roelofs AJ, Jauhiainen M, et al. Activation of gammadelta T cells by bisphosphonates. Adv Exp Med Biol 2010;658:11–20.
112. Dicuonzo G, Vincenzi B, Santini D, et al. Fever after zoledronic acid administration is due to increase in TNF-alpha and IL-6. J Interferon Cytokine Res 2003;23: 649–54.
113. Thompson K, Rogers MJ. Statins prevent bisphosphonate-induced gamma, delta-T-cell proliferation and activation in vitro. J Bone Miner Res 2004;19: 278–88.
114. Hewitt RE, Lissina A, Green AE, et al. The bisphosphonate acute phase response: rapid and copious production of proinflammatory cytokines by peripheral blood gd T cells in response to aminobisphosphonates is inhibited by statins. Clin Exp Immunol 2005;139:101–11.
115. Silverman SL, Kriegman A, Goncalves J, et al. Effect of acetaminophen and fluvastatin on post-dose symptoms following infusion of zoledronic acid. Osteoporos Int 2011;22:2337–45.
116. Thompson K, Keech F, McLernon DJ, et al. Fluvastatin does not prevent the acute-phase response to intravenous zoledronic acid in post-menopausal women. Bone 2011;49:140–5.
117. Srivastava T, Haney CJ, Alon US. Atorvastatin may have no effect on acute phase reaction in children after intravenous bisphosphonate infusion. J Bone Miner Res 2009;24:334–7.
118. Makras P, Anastasilakis AD, Polyzos SA, et al. No effect of rosuvastatin in the zoledronate-induced acute-phase response. Calcif Tissue Int 2011;88:402–8.
119. Tanvetyanon T, Stiff PJ. Management of the adverse effects associated with intravenous bisphosphonates. Ann Oncol 2006;17:897–907.
120. Macarol V, Fraunfelder FT. Pamidronate disodium and possible ocular adverse drug reactions. Am J Ophthalmol 1994;118:220–4.

121. McKague M, Jorgenson D, Buxton KA. Ocular side effects of bisphosphonates: a case report and literature review. Can Fam Physician 2010;56:1015–7.
122. Etminan M, Forooghian F, Maberley D. Inflammatory ocular adverse events with the use of oral bisphosphonates: a retrospective cohort study. CMAJ 2012;184: E431–4.
123. Mbekeani JN, Slamovits TL, Schwartz BH, et al. Ocular inflammation associated with alendronate therapy. Arch Ophthalmol 1999;117:837–8.
124. French DD, Margo CE. Postmarketing surveillance rates of uveitis and scleritis with bisphosphonates among a national veteran cohort. Retina 2008;28:889–93.
125. Wysowski DK, Chang JT. Alendronate and risedronate: reports of severe bone, joint, and muscle pain. Arch Intern Med 2005;165:346–7.
126. U.S. Food and Drug Administration. Bisphosphonates (marketed as Actonel, Actonel+Ca, Aredia, Boniva, Didronel, Fosamax, Fosamax+D, Reclast, Skelid, and Zometa) Information. Available at: http://www.fda.gov/drugs/drugsafety/ postmarketdrugsafetyinformationforpatientsandproviders/ucm101551.htm. Accessed September 17, 2012.
127. Caplan L, Pittman CB, Zeringue AL, et al. An observational study of musculoskeletal pain among patients receiving bisphosphonate therapy. Mayo Clin Proc 2010;85:341–8.
128. Body JJ, Pfister T, Bauss F. Preclinical perspectives on bisphosphonate renal safety. Oncologist 2005;10(Suppl 1):3–7.
129. Rosen LS, Gordon D, Kaminski M, et al. Long-term efficacy and safety of zoledronic acid compared with pamidronate disodium in the treatment of skeletal complications in patients with advanced multiple myeloma or breast carcinoma: a randomized, double-blind, multicenter, comparative trial. Cancer 2003;98:1735–44.
130. Berenson JR, Boccia R, Lopez T, et al. Results of a multicenter open-label randomized trial evaluating infusion duration of zoledronic acid in multiple myeloma patients (the ZMAX trial). J Support Oncol 2011;9:32–40.
131. Markowitz GS, Appel GB, Fine PL, et al. Collapsing focal segmental glomerulosclerosis following treatment with high-dose pamidronate. J Am Soc Nephrol 2001;12:1164–72.
132. U.S. Food and Drug Administration. FDA drug safety communication: new contraindication and updated warning on kidney impairment for Reclast (zoledronic acid). Available at: http://www.fda.gov/Drugs/DrugSafety/ucm270199. htm. Accessed September 17, 2012.
133. Miller PD. The kidney and bisphosphonates. Bone 2011;49:77–81.
134. Hirschberg R. Renal complications from bisphosphonate treatment. Curr Opin Support Palliat Care 2012;6:342–7.
135. Barri YM, Munshi NC, Sukumalchantra S, et al. Podocyte injury associated glomerulopathies induced by pamidronate. Kidney Int 2004;65:634–41.
136. Banerjee D, Asif A, Striker L, et al. Short-term, high-dose pamidronate-induced acute tubular necrosis: the postulated mechanisms of bisphosphonate nephrotoxicity. Am J Kidney Dis 2003;41:E18.
137. Yilmaz M, Taninmis H, Kara E, et al. Nephrotic syndrome after oral bisphosphonate (alendronate) administration in a patient with osteoporosis. Osteoporos Int 2012;23:2059–62.
138. Bodmer M, Amico P, Mihatsch MJ, et al. Focal segmental glomerulosclerosis associated with long-term treatment with zoledronate in a myeloma patient. Nephrol Dial Transplant 2007;22:2366–70.
139. Maalouf NM, Heller HJ, Odvina CV, et al. Bisphosphonate-induced hypocalcemia: report of 3 cases and review of literature. Endocr Pract 2006;12:48–53.

140. Chesnut CH 3rd, McClung MR, Ensrud KE, et al. Alendronate treatment of the postmenopausal osteoporotic woman: effect of multiple dosages on bone mass and bone remodeling. Am J Med 1995;99:144–52.

141. Harris ST, Gertz BJ, Genant HK, et al. The effect of short term treatment with alendronate on vertebral density and biochemical markers of bone remodeling in early postmenopausal women. J Clin Endocrinol Metab 1993;76:1399–406.

142. Mortensen L, Charles P, Bekker PJ, et al. Risedronate increases bone mass in an early postmenopausal population: two years of treatment plus one year of follow-up. J Clin Endocrinol Metab 1998;83:396–402.

143. Corporation NP. Highlights of prescribing information. East Hanover (NJ): Novartis; 2011. Available at: http://www.pharma.us.novartis.com/product/pi/pdf/reclast.pdf.

144. Chennuru S, Koduri J, Baumann MA. Risk factors for symptomatic hypocalcaemia complicating treatment with zoledronic acid. Intern Med J 2008;38:635–7.

145. Tsourdi E, Rachner TD, Gruber M, et al. Seizures associated with zoledronic acid for osteoporosis. J Clin Endocrinol Metab 2011;96:1955–9.

146. Papapoulos SE, Harinck HI, Bijvoet OL, et al. Effects of decreasing serum calcium on circulating parathyroid hormone and vitamin D metabolites in normocalcaemic and hypercalcaemic patients treated with APD. Bone Miner 1986;1:69–78.

147. Quandt SA, Thompson DE, Schneider DL, et al. Effect of alendronate on vertebral fracture risk in women with bone mineral density T scores of-1.6 to -2.5 at the femoral neck: the Fracture Intervention Trial. Mayo Clin Proc 2005;80:343–9.

148. Watts NB, Diab DL. Long-term use of bisphosphonates in osteoporosis. J Clin Endocrinol Metab 2010;95:1555–65.

149. Watts NB, Bilezikian JP, Camacho PM, et al. American Association of Clinical Endocrinologists Medical Guidelines for Clinical Practice for the diagnosis and treatment of postmenopausal osteoporosis. Endocr Pract 2010;16(Suppl 3):1–37.

Nonserious Infections
Should There Be Cause for Serious Concerns?

Kathryn H. Dao, MD[a],*, Morley Herbert, PhD[b], Nadia Habal, MD[c],
John J. Cush, MD[a]

KEYWORDS

- Nonserious infections • Anti-TNF • Adalimumab • Etanercept • Infliximab • Safety
- Rheumatoid arthritis

KEY POINTS

- RA patients commonly encounter nonserious infections (NSIE) as upper respiratory tract infection, minor skin/soft tissue infections, urinary tract infections.
- Anti-TNF therapy can increase the risk for NSIE.
- NSIE are likely self-limited and may not progress to more serious infections.

INTRODUCTION

Although the use of biologic agents is becoming more commonplace in clinical practice, concern for safety has been mounting. The tumor necrosis factor-alpha inhibitors (TNFi) are the most commonly prescribed biologic agents for the treatment of immune-mediated inflammatory diseases (IMID). Five TNFi are commercially available in the United States for clinical use: adalimumab (ADA), etanercept (ETN), infliximab (INF), golimumab, and certolizumab. Many studies have published on adverse events (AE) associated with these biologics, with the vast majority focusing on serious infectious events (SIE), which have been defined as infections that are life-threatening or those that require hospitalization or intravenous (IV) antibiotics.[1–7] However, very limited data are available on the most prevalent AE encountered by patients who are routinely treated with TNFi: the nonserious infections (NSIE). NSIE may include upper respiratory tract infections (URI), influenza (flu) syndromes, urinary tract infections (UTI), and skin/soft tissue infections (SSI). These infections account for more

Disclosures: Dr Cush: Clinical Investigator for Genentech, Pfizer, UCB, Celgene, CORRONA; consultant to Centocor, UCB, Wyeth, Amgen, Roche, BMS, Savient. Dr Dao: Clinical Investigator for UCB, Celgene, Amgen, Abbott, Centocor, Genentech, speaker for Lilly, National Advisory Board for GSK.
[a] Baylor Research Institute, 9900 North Central Expressway, Suite #550, Dallas, TX 75229, USA;
[b] Medical City Dallas Hospital, 7777 Forest Lane, Suite C-740, Dallas, TX 75230, USA; [c] Northern Virginia Arthritis, 101 South Whiting Street, Suite 105, Alexandria, VA 22304, USA
* Corresponding author.
E-mail address: daokathryn@yahoo.com

than 50 million outpatient or emergency department visits annually, with an estimated economic burden of more than $40 billion in direct and indirect costs. [8–13] **Fig. 1** shows the estimated annual socioeconomic burden of NSIE in the general US population.

It is unclear how TNFi impact the outcome of these common infections. Are frequencies and types of infections different in patients receiving TNFi? Do NSIE progress to serious infections in these patients (should TNFi therapy be interrupted when patients develop one of these infections)? Do dosages or the frequency of TNFi exposure matter? Are certain TNFi more likely to cause NSIE? In an attempt to answer these questions, the authors conducted a meta-analysis on NSIE of published, large, randomized, double-blinded, placebo-controlled trials (RDBPCT) of the top 3 prescribed TNFi, ADA, ETN, and INF, in patients with IMID.

MATERIALS AND METHODS
Definition

In industry-sponsored studies, the regulatory definition of SIE would be a serious AE (SAE) of an infectious nature. SAE include events that are life threatening; require serious interventions; and result in hospitalization, disability, or death. In publications and medical practice, SIE also include opportunistic infections or infections requiring IV antibiotics or hospitalization. A standard definition of NSIE does not exist. For the purpose of this study, NSIE was predefined as an infection not requiring IV antibiotics or hospitalization and not otherwise classified as a SIE by the study investigators. Infections falling into this category would include URI, pharyngitis, rhinitis, sinusitis, bronchitis, UTI, flu, SSI, and mild cases of cellulitis that do not require IV antibiotics or hospitalization.

Study Selection Criteria

A systemic literature search was performed in PubMed, OVID Medline, and Cochrane Database between 1966-2010 using the following search strings: biologics, tumor necrosis factor inhibitor, tumor necrosis receptor, adalimumab, etanercept, infliximab, inflammatory arthritis, rheumatoid arthritis (RA), psoriasis, psoriatic arthritis, ankylosing spondylitis, Crohn's disease, inflammatory bowel disease (IBD), ulcerative colitis limits set for English language, and randomized controlled trials involving humans of adult age. For inclusion in the meta-analysis, the randomized controlled trial (RCT) must have (1) at least 50 patients exposed to TNFi with matched controls, (2) a follow-up of at least 12 weeks, and (3) documentation of the number or rate of NSIE. Excluded are trials that involve switching, lack of or inadequate documentation of NSIE, trials involving off-label use of the drugs, and trials involving use of

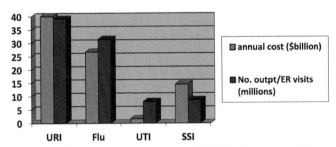

Fig. 1. Estimated annual socioeconomic burden of NSIE in the general US population. ER, emergency room. (*Data from* Refs.[8–12])

combination biologics. Trials that document NSIE events exceeding the number of patients and in which events per patient-year were not defined were also excluded because these publications did not disclose the number of patients who experienced an NSIE event. For trials with interim analyses, the most recent data reported were included in the analysis. Trials with extended follow-up periods were evaluated up to the point when controls were given an active drug. All studies that were identified for possible inclusion in the analysis were reviewed in detail by 2 rheumatologists and a statistician for inclusion or exclusion; trials in which no general agreement was reached were adjudicated by a third rheumatologist.

Statistical Method

Statistical analysis was conducted using the Comprehensive Meta Analysis program (version 2.2) with the random-effects model. Risk ratios (RR) were derived by comparing the NSIE rate for each TNFi against placebo or the background disease-modifying antirheumatic drug (DMARD) rate. Subset analyses were performed examining NSIE relationships with dosing regimens and timing intervals. Low/standard-dosage drug exposure was also predefined as follows: ADA 40 mg or less every 2 weeks, ETN 50 mg or less every week, and INF less than 5 mg/kg every 8 weeks. Any regimen that exceeded the predefined low/standard-dosage exposure amount was considered a high-dosage exposure. Analyses were conducted (1) to determine rates of NSIE in TNFi-exposed groups compared with control groups, (2) to see if the dosing regimen influenced the outcome, (3) to see if the NSIE rates changed over time, and (4) to evaluate types of NSIE seen with each agent.

RESULTS

Using the previously mentioned search strings, 293 RCT studies were identified. Thirty-four studies met preset inclusion criteria: 11 ADA trials,[14–24] 13 ETN trials,[25–38] and 10 INF trials[39–48]; however, 1 trial[24] was not included in the meta-analysis because only events per patient-year were reported. The number of NSIE, types of events, and number of patients who experienced the NSIE were not listed separately, interfering with data interpretation. **Fig. 2** details the selection process for this systematic review. This meta-analysis of 33 trials encompasses 14 553 patients and more than 7910 patient-years of follow-up. **Table 1** summarizes the details of these trials.

Analyses were conducted evaluating the risk of NSIE associated with each TNFi. NSIE RR were calculated by comparing NSIE rates in those exposed to the specified TNFi with NSIE rates in control arms (**Fig. 3**). For patients exposed to ADA, the RR was 1.194 (95% confidence interval [CI] 1.085–1.315, $P<.001$), for ETN the RR was 1.028 (95% CI 0.909–1.162, $P = .665$), and for INF the RR was 1.194 (95% CI 1.014–1.406, $P = .034$). Events per patient-year varied widely among the studies. On average, ADA yielded 1.1 events per patient-year, ETN 0.8 events per patient-year, INF 3.0 events per patient-year, while for controls there were 0.76 events per patient-year. The anti-TNF therapy in RA with concomitant therapy (ATTRACT) trial (see **Table 1**) disproportionately skews the INF event rate by reporting 40 NSIE per patient-year in the INF group compared with 0.71 events per patient-year in the control group.[46] All trials noted that respiratory tract infections (RTI), including URI, rhinitis, and sinusitis, were the most commonly reported NSIE, consisting of 65% of NSIE infections. Flu syndromes, UTI, and skin infections each contributed to 10% to 15% of NSIE (**Fig. 4**). The reported frequency of NSIE-related study withdrawal was not different compared with placebo or background DMARD (data not shown). Next, the effect of the dosages was evaluated to see if

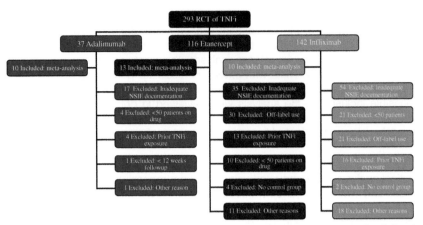

Fig. 2. Study selection for meta-analysis. Other reasons for exclusion were the following: study was an interim analysis, TNFi was not the intended study drug, trial was an open-label extension study, NSIE events exceed number of patients, combination biologic therapy was used, or data were uninterpretable.

this had an influence on the frequency of NSIE. When studies were segregated according to the amount of drug exposure, the risk for NSIE was significantly increased at both low and higher dosages for ADA and INF but not for ETN (**Figs. 5** and **6**). A dose-related increase in NSIE was seen with ADA only (**Fig. 7**). Finally, an evaluation of the rate of NSIE with the length of the study was also conducted to see if the number of NSIE increased or decreased with the duration of drug exposure and the length of the clinical trial. The number of events did not seem to increase with time for all 3 TNFi (**Fig. 8**).

DISCUSSION

TNF-alpha serves important roles in host defense (ie, activating monocytes/macrophages/T and B cells, inducing proinflammatory cytokines, and promoting chemotaxis and the migration of cells), all of which help to facilitate actions to control infection.[49] With increased numbers of prescriptions for TNFi being written every year and with patients exposed to the drug over extended periods of time, concerns for safety have mounted. Many studies have focused on serious infections, neglecting the most common infections. To the best of the authors' knowledge, this is the only systematic review of RCTs evaluating the risk of NSIE in patients exposed to TNFi. Published RCTs have recorded NSIE frequencies to be 10 to 20 times that of SIE in patients treated with TNFi.[14–48] Previous studies of registries and databanks confirmed that these infections are common.[3,50] Dixon and colleagues[50] analyzed a cohort of 13 634 elderly patients with RA (28 695 person-years of follow-up); the NSIE incidence rate was estimated to be 47.5 per 100 patient-years. The investigators' meta-analysis revealed that these events are likely more common in patients with IMID treated with biologics. Despite the frequency of these events, little is known about their impact and outcome. This meta-analysis compared the rate and types of NSIE of the 3 most commonly used TNFi: ADA, ETN, and INF. These results indicate that patients exposed to ADA and INF may have a slightly increased risk for developing NSIE compared with ETN. ADA and INF are estimated to confer a 20% higher risk for

Table 1
Summary of randomized controlled trials of tumor necrosis factor inhibitors in immune-mediated inflammatory diseases

Reference	Disease	Comparator	Anti-TNF Drug	Concentration	Dosing Interval	Hi/Lo Dosage	Study Period	Number of Study Patients	Study NSIE	Number Control Patients	Number Control NSIE	Study py	Control py	Study E/py	Control E/py	Notes
ADA (Humira)																
Saurat et al,[14] 2008	Psoriasis	Placebo	ADA	40 mg	q 2 wk	Lo	16 wk	107	87	53	42	32.9	16.3	2.64	2.58	
Menter et al,[15] 2008	Psoriasis	Placebo	ADA	40 mg	q 2 wk	Lo	16 wk	814	230	398	85	250.5	122.5	0.92	0.69	
Genovese et al,[16] 2007	Psoriatic arthritis	Placebo	ADA	40 mg	q 2 wk	Lo	12 wk	51	15	49	9	11.8	11.3	1.27	0.8	
van der Heijde et al,[17] 2006	Ankylosing spondylitis	Placebo	ADA	40 mg	q 2 wk	Lo	24 wk	208	66	107	22	96.0	44.3	0.69	0.5	
Breedveld et al,[24] 2006	RA	MTX	ADA	40 mg	q 2 wk	Lo	104 wk	268	—	257	—	482.0	429.0	1.2	1.17	Had to exclude the trial from analysis because data only present as events per pats without details how many pats had the events
Mease et al,[18] 2005	Psoriatic Arthritis	Placebo	ADA	40 mg	q 2 wk	Lo	24 wk	151	34	162	39	69.7	74.8	0.49	0.52	
Keystone et al,[19] 2004	RA	Placebo	ADA	40 mg / 20 mg	q 2 wk / q 2 wk	Std/lo / Std/lo	52 wk / —	207 / 212	123 / 142	200 / —	95 / —	179.2 / 186.7	161.3 / —	0.69 / 0.76	0.59 / —	

(continued on next page)

Table 1
(continued)

Reference	Disease	Comparator	Anti-TNF Drug	Concentration	Dosing Interval	Hi/Lo Dosage	Study Period	Number of Study Patients	Study NSIE	Number Control Patients	Number Control NSIE	Study py	Control py	Study E/py	Control E/py	Notes
van de Putte et al,[20] 2004	RA	Placebo	ADA	20 mg	q 2 wk	Std/lo	26 wk	106	11	110	12	53.0	55.0	0.21	0.22	
				20 mg	1/wk	Std/lo	—	112	21	—	—	56.0	—	0.38	—	
				40 mg	q 2 wk	Std/lo	—	113	21	—	—	56.5	—	0.37	—	
				40 mg	1/wk	Hi	—	103	22	—	—	51.5	—	0.43	—	
Weinblatt et al,[21] 2003	RA	Placebo	ADA	20 mg	q 2 wk	Std/lo	24 wk	69	38	62	23	27.4	21.0	1.39	1.1	
				40 mg	q 2 wk	Std/lo	—	67	37	—	—	28.2	—	1.31	—	
				80 mg	q 2 wk	Hi	—	73	38	—	—	31.4	—	1.21	—	
van de Putte et al,[22] 2003	RA	Placebo	ADA	20 mg	1/wk	Std/lo	12 wk	72	11	70	7	16.6	16.2	0.66	0.43	
				40 mg	1/wk	Hi	12 wk	70	11	—	—	16.2	—	0.68	—	
				80 mg	1/wk	Hi	12 wk	72	7	—	—	16.6	—	0.42	—	
Furst et al,[23] 2003	RA	Placebo	ADA	40 mg	q 2 wk	Std/lo	24 wk	318	162	318	151	146.8	146.8	1.1	1.03	
							358 wk	3193		1786		1809.0	1098.5			
ETN (Enbrel)																
Emery et al,[25] 2008	RA	MTX	ETN	50 mg	1/wk	Hi	52 wk	274	55	268	53	274	268.0	0.2	0.2	
Weisman et al,[26] 2007	RA	Placebo	ETN	25 mg	2/wk	Hi	16 wk	266	98	269	107	81.8	82.8	1.2	—	

Study	Disease	Control	Drug	Dose	Freq	Level	Duration	N	N	N	N					Comments
Tyring et al,[27] 2007	Psoriasis	Placebo	ETN	50 mg	2/wk	Hi	96 wk (12 then open label)	598	—	306	—	908.9	65.9	1.03	1.29	Open-label so corrected for exposure, only event/pat-y are usable, this was an f/u to the Tyring 2007, open labeled (unable to use)
van der Heijde et al,[28] 2006	Ankylosing spondylitis	Placebo	ETN	50 mg	1/wk	Hi	12 wk	155	34	51	12	35.8	11.8	0.95	1.02	
				25 mg	2/wk	Hi	12 wk	150	32	—	—	34.6	—	0.92	—	
Tyring et al,[29] 2006	Psoriasis	Placebo	ETN	50 mg	2/wk	Hi	12 wk	312	87	306	70	72	70.6	1.21	0.99	Follow-up data is in Tyring 2007
van der Heijde et al,[30] 2006	RA	MTX	ETN	25 mg	2/wk	Lo	104 wk	231	162	228	157	419.0	380.0	0.39	0.41	Cannot use ETN-alone group, no control
Papp et al,[31] 2005	Psoriasis	Placebo	ETN	25 mg	2/wk	Lo	12 wk	196	35	193	28	45.2	44.5	0.77	0.63	
				50 mg	2/wk	Hi	—	194	33	—	—	44.8	—	0.74	—	
Keystone et al,[32] 2004	RA	MTX	ETN	50 mg	1/wk	Std/lo	8 wk	214	6	53	7	32.9	8.2	0.18	0.85	
				25 mg	2/wk	Std/lo	8 wk	153	9	—	—	23.5	—	0.38	—	
Mease et al,[33] 2004	Psoriatic arthritis	Placebo	ETN	25 mg	2/wk	Std/lo	24 wk	101	33	104	38	46.6	48.0	0.71	0.79	
Leonardi et al,[34] 2003	Psoriasis	Placebo	ETN	25 mg	1/wk	Std/lo	12 wk	160	16	166	20	36.9	38.3	0.43	0.52	
				25 mg	2/wk	Std/lo	12 wk	162	15	—	—	37.4	—	0.4	—	
				50 mg	2/wk	Hi	12 wk	164	9	—	—	37.8	—	0.24	—	

(continued on next page)

Table 1
(continued)

Reference	Disease	Comparator	Anti-TNF Drug	Concentration	Dosing Interval	Hi/Lo Dosage	Study Period	Number of Study Patients	Study NSIE	Number Control Patients	Number Control NSIE	Study py	Control py	Study E/py	Control E/py	Notes
Davis et al,[35] 2003	Ankylosing spondylitis	Placebo	ETN	25 mg	2/wk	Std/lo	24 wk	138	41	139	35	63.7	64.2	0.64	0.55	
Gottlieb et al,[36] 2003	Psoriasis	Topicals	ETN	25 mg	2/wk	Std/lo	24 wk	57	28	55	13	23.6	14.5	1.57	1.24	
Bathon et al,[37] 2000	RA	MTX	ETN	10 mg 25 mg	2/wk	Std/lo	52 wk	208 207	163 177	217	197	208.0 207.0	217.0 —	0.78 0.86	0.91 —	
Moreland et al,[38] 1999	RA	Placebo	ETN	10 mg 25 mg	2/wk 2/wk	Lo Lo	26 wk —	76 78 4094	46 60	80 — 2435	61 —	31 33.0 2697.5	22.0 — 1335.8	1.47 1.82	1.86 —	
INF (Remicade)																
Westhovens et al,[39] 2006	RA	Placebo	INF	3 mg/kg 10 mg/kg	0/2/6/14 wk —	Std/lo Hi	22 wk —	360 361	59 84	361 —	64 —	152.3 152.7	152.7 —	0.42 0.55	0.42 —	
Reich et al,[40] 2005	Psoriasis	Placebo	INF	5 mg/kg	0/2/6 q 8 wk	Hi	24 wk	298	95	76	27	137.5	35.1	0.69	0.77	
Kavanaugh et al,[41] 2005	Psoriatic arthritis	Placebo	INF	5 mg/kg	0/2/6/14/22 wk	Hi	24 wk	150	31	97	22	69.2	44.8	0.45	0.49	
Antoni et al,[42] 2005	Psoriatic arthritis	Placebo	INF	5 mg/kg	0/2/6/14 wk	Hi	16 wk	52	8	51	15	16.0	15.7	0.5	0.96	

Study	Disease	Comparator	Drug	Dose	Schedule	Level	f/u									Notes
van der Heijde et al,[43] 2005	Ankylosing spondylitis	Placebo	INF	5 mg/kg	0/2/6/12/18 wk	Hi	24 wk	202	86	75	27	93.2	34.6	0.92	0.78	
Rutgeerts et al,[44] 2005	Ulcerative colitis	Placebo	INF	5 mg/kg	0/2/6 q 8 wk	Hi	54 wk (I)	121	50	121	42	125.7	125.7	0.4	0.33	
				10 mg/kg	0/2/6 q 8 wk	Hi	54 wk (I)	122	52	—	—	126.7	—	0.41	—	
				5 mg/kg	0/2/6 q 8 wk	Hi	30 wk (II)	121	31	123	28	69.8	71.0	0.44	0.39	
				10 mg/kg	0/2/6 q 8 wk	Hi	30 wk (II)	120	31	—	—	69.2	—	0.45	—	
St Clair et al,[45] 2004	RA	Placebo	INF	3 mg/kg	0/2/6 q 8 wk	Std/lo	54 wk	372	173	291	101	386.3	302.1	0.45	0.33	
				6 mg/kg	0/2/6 q 8 wk	Hi	—	377	184	—	—	391.5	—	0.47	—	
Maini et al,[46] 1999	RA	Placebo	INF	3 mg/kg	q r8 wk	Std/lo	30 wk	89	46	86	29	51.3	0.9	40.7	0.71	Corrected pat-y for controls; 35% dropout
				3 mg/kg	q r4 wk	Hi	—	86	35	—	—	49.6	0.71	—	—	
				10 mg/kg	q 8 wk	Hi	—	87	51	—	—	50.2	1.02	—	—	
				10 mg/kg	q 4 wk	Hi	—	80	55	—	—	46.2	1.19	—	—	
Present et al,[47] 1999	Crohn	Placebo	INF	5 mg/kg	0/2/6 wk	Hi	18 wk	31	1	31	2	10.7	10.7	0.093	0.19	
				10 mg/kg	0/2/6 wk	Hi	—	32	5	—	—	11.1	—	0.45	—	
Maini et al,[48] 1998	RA	MTX	INF	Various	Various	Hi	26 wk	87	28	14	3	43.5	7.0	0.64	0.43	Poor paper combines all groups
								3148	1326			2052.7	803.22			

Abbreviations: f/u, follow-up; Pats, patients; Pat-y, patient-years; Std, standard.

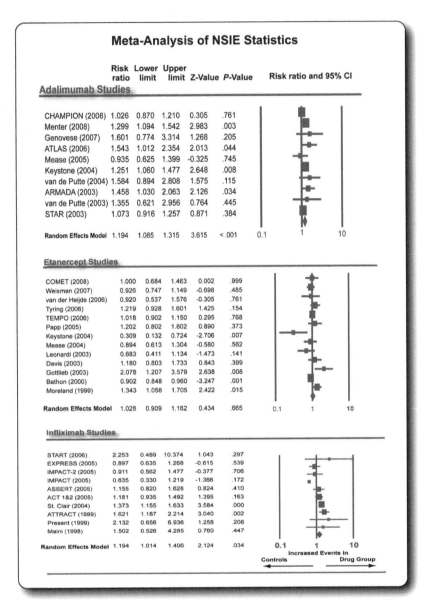

Fig. 3. Calculated NSIE RR for ADA, ETN, and INF. CI, confidence interval.

NSIE compared with ETN and DMARD/placebo. These findings are consistent with other studies that have suggested that the monoclonal anti–TNF-alpha antibodies (mTNF-a Ab), ADA, and INF may cause higher rates of Herpes zoster, tuberculosis, and nontuberculosis opportunistic infections[51–54] compared with the soluble TNF receptor antagonist, ETN. It is unknown if differences in incidences of infections seen among ADA, ETN, and INF are related to their construct, half-life, or binding affinities. Mitoma and colleagues[55] demonstrated through in vivo studies that the

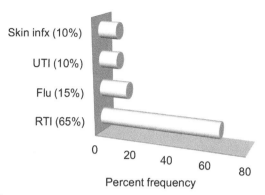

Fig. 4. Types and frequency of nonserious infections associated with TNFi use.

mTNF-a Ab have the ability to induce complement-dependent cytotoxicity, antibody-dependent cell-mediated cytotoxicity (ADCC), and outside-to-inside reverse signaling for apoptosis/cell cycle arrest, whereas ETN had only ADCC activity but lacked other activities, hence, making it less efficient in destroying TNF-producing cells. Although the NSIE risk is small but significantly increased with ADA and INF, this risk persists despite the dosing regimen. With ADA, the risk for NSIE is also significantly increased when dosages of more than 40 mg every 2 weeks were used. These findings are similar to prior studies evaluating SIE, which found that higher dosages of TNFi may carry higher risks for SIE.[39,56] Most NSIE were related to RTI as nasopharyngitis, rhinitis, and sinusitis; but 35% of NSIE were related to flu syndromes, UTI, and SSI. In the authors' study, it seemed that the rate of NSIE remained steady during the duration of drug exposure when compared with controls. The reported frequency of NSIE-related study withdrawal was not different compared with placebo or background DMARD. Most study withdrawals that were reported in the trials were related to SAE/SIE, but it is not known whether the SIE started with an NSIE or if patients had multiple NSIE before developing the SIE that terminated them from the study. Many investigators acknowledged that the survivability of the drug is not just related to drug efficacy but also to lower AE rates (eg, patients are more likely to stay on a drug if they do not experience a side effect that would force them to stop the drug); hence, the rate of SIE may seem to decrease with long-term TNFi use because those who experience SIE that lead them to discontinue the drug would not have been included in the long-term analysis.[2,57,58] The Swiss RA cohort study examined reasons for the discontinuation and retention of the drug over time and noted that AEs were responsible for treatment discontinuation in 48.7% of cases.[59] In the authors' study, NSIE rates remain steady despite the long-term use of these medications, perhaps suggesting that these infections may not turn into something more serious that would require discontinuation of therapy. Events per patient-year of NSIE vary widely among the studies, which may indicate a variance in reporting such events in clinical trials; in addition, many studies have a lower cut-off for reporting NSIE, often < 5% or patients or 10%. These contributions are missing from the analyzed data.

Several limitations are acknowledged in this meta-analysis including that each type of IMID were not represented equally in the each of the TNFi. It is unclear whether certain patient populations have greater rates of NSIE. The Safety Assessment of Biologic Therapy (SABER) project reported that SIE rates were higher in patients with IBD and RA compared with psoriasis and the spondyloarthritides.[60] Patients with IBD are

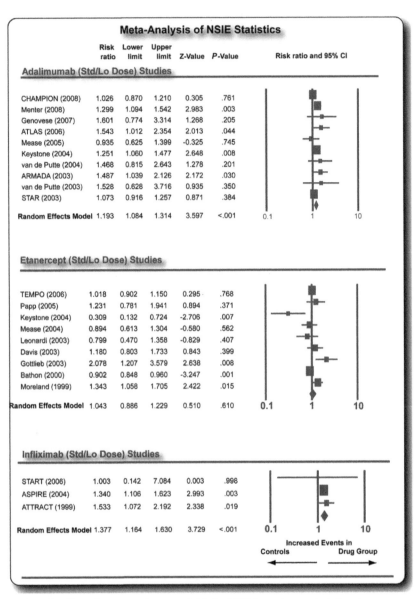

Fig. 5. Standard/low-dosage regimen and risk for NSIE. Low dosage is defined as exposure to ADA 40 mg or less every 2 weeks, for ETN 50 mg or less every week, for INF less than 5 mg/kg every 8 weeks.

prescribed ADA and INF, which is approved by the Food and Drug Administration for these diseases, but ETN is not. The authors' analysis included patients with IBD in the INF group; thus, rates of NSIE may have been higher with this drug because of the inclusion of IBD in the analysis. In addition, a greater number of ETN studies were represented compared with ADA and INF (13 vs 10 and 10, respectively), which could

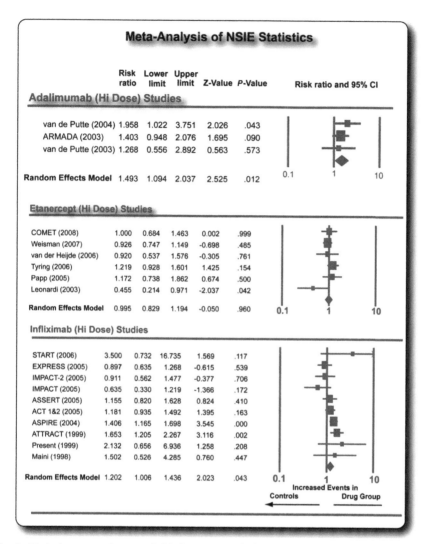

Fig. 6. High-dosage regimen and risk for NSIE. High dosage is defined as exposure to ADA more than 40 mg every 2 weeks, for ETN more than 50 mg every week, for INF 5 mg/kg or more every 8 weeks.

have leveled the effects of NSIE reported for ETN. Furthermore, the studies used for the meta-analysis were heterogeneous; they differ in IMID, comorbidities, length of follow-up, use of background DMARD, and steroid exposure. Dixon and colleagues found that the risk for NSIE was higher in patients exposed to a glucocorticoid versus those who were unexposed (52.4 vs 38.8 per 100 person-years, respectively) and noted that the risk for NSIE was present at all dosages of glucocorticoids (including <5 mg/d) and was higher than that seen for methotrexate (adjusted RR 1.00; 0.95–1.04). The amount of steroids patients were exposed to during the RCTs was variable and may have contributed to an increased number of NSIE reported. Finally, the most

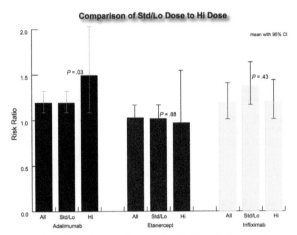

Fig. 7. Comparing standard/low-dose regimen with higher-dosing regimen and risk for NSIE.

important limitation of this study was that there was no standard definition of NSIE; studies had no preset protocol on how to document these infections. NSIE may not be reported by patients or erroneously recorded such that minor signs/symptoms that are not infection related may be mistaken for an infectious event (eg, allergic rhinitis mistaken for infectious rhinitis and asymptomatic pyuria recorded as a UTI). Many studies were not powered to detect NSIE, although these events are common. Because there is no preset protocol on how to document or manage these infections, NSIE may be underreported or overreported and inappropriately recorded.

Despite the frequency of NSIE, it appears that these types of infections do not progress to more serious infections suggested by the rate of SIE in patients exposed to TNFi were similar to controls and that rates of NSIE remain steady over time as rates of SIE seem to decrease. Clinicians vary widely in their empiric approach to treat these events; just as likely, clinical researchers vary in their approach to treating these NSIE during the clinical trials. Does one suspend TNFi use during these infections? Should antibiotics be given every time one of these events occur to prevent an SIE? Based on

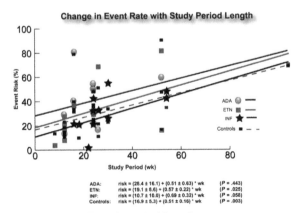

Fig. 8. Change in event rate with study period length.

the results of the RDBPCT, rates of SIE are not statistically increased in patients who were given TNFi compared with controls; it is unlikely that the study drug was held or antibiotics prescribed given the frequency of NSIE during any given trial. Plausible verdicts are the following: (1) TNFi therapy does not need to be suspended during an NSIE and (2) antibiotics are not routinely necessary to treat an NSIE. Real-world data from registries would be helpful to see if these hypotheses are cogent.

SUMMARY

NSIE (eg, RTI, flu syndromes, UTI, and skin infections) are common and seem to be increased in patients receiving TNFi. The risk for NSIE is estimated to be 20% higher in patients receiving ADA and INF independent of the dosing regimen based on the authors' meta-analysis of RDBPCT in patients with IMID. It is likely that NSIE tend to be self-limiting because SIE do not seem to be significantly higher in patients receiving TNFi compared with controls in most RCTs. However, further studies are needed to examine these types of infections, to evaluate the practice of continuing or suspending TNFi therapy in the face of NSIE, and to assess if certain patient populations are more susceptible to developing these types of infections.

REFERENCES

1. Dixon WG, Watson K, Lunt M, et al. Rates of serious infection, including site specific and bacterial intracellular infection, in rheumatoid arthritis patients receiving anti-TNF necrosis factor therapy. Arthritis Rheum 2006;54(8):2368–76.
2. Wolfe F, Caplan L, Michaud K. Treatment for rheumatoid arthritis and the risk of hospitalization for pneumonia. Arthritis Rheum 2006;54(2):628–34.
3. Listing J, Strangfeld A, Kary S, et al. Infections in patients with rheumatoid arthritis treated with biologic agents. Arthritis Rheum 2005;52(11):3403–12.
4. Doran M, Crowson C, Pond G, et al. Frequency of infection in patients with rheumatoid arthritis compared with controls: a population based study. Arthritis Rheum 2002;46(9):2287–93.
5. Bongartz T, Sutton A, Sweeting M, et al. Anti-TNF antibody therapy in rheumatoid arthritis and the risk of serious infections and malignancies: systematic review and meta-analysis of rare harmful effects in randomized controlled trials. JAMA 2006;295(19):2275–85.
6. Fernandez-Nebro A, Irigoyen M, Urena I, et al. Effectiveness, predictive response factors, and safety of anti-tumor necrosis factor (TNF) therapies in anti-TNF-naïve rheumatoid arthritis. J Rheumatol 2007;34(12):2334–42.
7. Kroesen S, Widmer AF, Tyndall A, et al. Serious bacterial infections in patients with rheumatoid arthritis under anti-TNF-a therapy. Rheumatology 2003;42: 617–21.
8. Poole MD, Portugal LG. Treatment of rhinosinusitis in the outpatient setting. Am J Med 2005;118:45S–50S.
9. Fendrick AM, Monto AS, Nightingale B, et al. The economic burden of non-influenza-related viral respiratory tract infection in the United States. Arch Intern Med 2003;163:487–94.
10. Foxman B. Epidemiology of urinary tract infections: incidence, morbidity, and economic costs. Am J Med 2002;113(Suppl 1A):5S–13S.
11. Keating KN, Perfetto EM, Subedi P. Economic burden of uncomplicated urinary tract infections: direct, indirect and intangible costs. Expert Rev Pharmacoecon Outcomes Res 2005;5(4):457–66.

12. Molinari NA, Ortega-Sanchez IR, Messonnier ML, et al. The annual impact of seasonal influenza in the US: measuring disease burden and costs. Vaccine 2007;25(27):5086–96.
13. Pallin DJ, Egan DJ, Pelletier AJ, et al. Increased US emergency department visits for skin and soft tissue infections, and changes in antibiotic choices, during the emergence of community-associated methicillin-resistant *Staphylococcus aureus*. Ann Emerg Med 2008;51(3):291–8 [Epub 2008 Jan 28].
14. Saurat JH, Stingl G, Dubertret L, et al, CHAMPION Study Investigators. Efficacy and safety results from the randomized controlled comparative study of adalimumab vs. methotrexate vs. placebo in patients with psoriasis (CHAMPION). Br J Dermatol 2008;158:558–66.
15. Menter A, Tyring SK, Gordon K, et al. Adalimumab therapy for moderate to severe psoriasis: a randomized, controlled phase III trial. J Am Acad Dermatol 2008;58: 106–15.
16. Genovese MC, Mease PJ, Thomson GT, et al, M02-570 Study Group. Safety and efficacy of adalimumab in treatment of patients with psoriatic arthritis who had failed disease modifying antirheumatic drug therapy. J Rheumatol 2007;34: 1040–50.
17. van der Heijde D, Kivitz A, Schiff MH, et al, ATLAS Study Group. Efficacy and safety of adalimumab in patients with ankylosing spondylitis: results of a multi-center, randomized, double-blind, placebo-controlled trial. Arthritis Rheum 2006;54:2136–46.
18. Mease PJ, Gladman DD, Ritchlin CT, et al, Adalimumab Effectiveness in Psoriatic Arthritis Trial Study Group. Adalimumab for the treatment of patients with moder-ately to severely active psoriatic arthritis: results of a double-blind, randomized, placebo-controlled trial. Arthritis Rheum 2005;52:3279–89.
19. Keystone EC, Kavanaugh AF, Sharp JT, et al. Radiographic, clinical, and func-tional outcomes of treatment with adalimumab (a human anti-tumor necrosis factor monoclonal antibody) in patients with active rheumatoid arthritis receiving concomitant methotrexate therapy: a randomized, placebo-controlled, 52-week trial. Arthritis Rheum 2004;50:1400–11.
20. Van de Putte LB, Atkins C, Malaise M, et al. Efficacy and safety of adalimumab as monotherapy in patients with rheumatoid arthritis for whom previous disease modi-fying antirheumatic drug treatment has failed. Ann Rheum Dis 2004;63:508–16.
21. Weinblatt ME, Keystone EC, Furst DE, et al. Adalimumab, a fully human anti-tumor necrosis factor alpha monoclonal antibody, for the treatment of rheumatoid arthritis in patients taking concomitant methotrexate: the ARMADA trial. Arthritis Rheum 2003;48:35–45.
22. Van de Putte LB, Rau R, Breedveld FC, et al. Efficacy and safety of the fully human anti-tumour necrosis factor alpha monoclonal antibody adalimumab (D2E7) in DMARD refractory patients with rheumatoid arthritis: a 12 week, phase II study. Ann Rheum Dis 2003;62:1168–77.
23. Furst DE, Schiff MH, Fleischmann RM, et al. Adalimumab, a fully human anti tumor necrosis factor-alpha monoclonal antibody, and concomitant standard anti-rheumatic therapy for the treatment of rheumatoid arthritis: results of STAR (Safety Trial of Adalimumab in Rheumatoid Arthritis). J Rheumatol 2003;30:2563–71.
24. Breedveld FC, Weisman MH, Kavanaugh AF, et al. The PREMIER study: a multi-center, randomized, double-blind clinical trial of combination therapy with adali-mumab plus methotrexate versus methotrexate alone or adalimumab alone in patients with early, aggressive rheumatoid arthritis who had not had previous methotrexate treatment. Arthritis Rheum 2006;54:26–37.

25. Emery P, Breedveld FC, Hall S, et al. Comparison of methotrexate monotherapy with a combination of methotrexate and etanercept in active, early, moderate to severe rheumatoid arthritis (COMET): a randomised, double-blind, parallel treatment trial. Lancet 2008;372(9636):375–82.

26. Weisman MH, Paulus HE, Burch FX, et al. A placebo-controlled, randomized, double-blinded study evaluating the safety of etanercept in patients with rheumatoid arthritis and concomitant comorbid diseases. Rheumatology (Oxford) 2007; 46:1122–5.

27. Tyring S, Gordon KB, Poulin Y, et al. Long-term safety and efficacy of 50 mg of etanercept twice weekly in patients with psoriasis. Arch Dermatol 2007;143: 719–26.

28. Van der Heijde D, Da Silva JC, Dougados M, et al, Etanercept Study 314 Investigators. Etanercept 50 mg once weekly is as effective as 25 mg twice weekly in patients with ankylosing spondylitis. Ann Rheum Dis 2006;65:1572–7.

29. Tyring S, Gottlieb A, Papp K, et al. Etanercept and clinical outcomes, fatigue, and depression in psoriasis: double-blind placebo-controlled randomised phase III trial. Lancet 2006;367:29–35.

30. van der Heijde D, Klareskog L, Rodriguez-Valverde V, et al, TEMPO Study Investigators. Comparison of etanercept and methotrexate, alone and combined, in the treatment of rheumatoid arthritis: two-year clinical and radiographic results from the TEMPO study, a double-blind, randomized trial. Arthritis Rheum 2006; 54:1063–74.

31. Papp KA, Tyring S, Lahfa M, et al, Etanercept Psoriasis Study Group. A global phase III randomized controlled trial of etanercept in psoriasis: safety, efficacy, and effect of dose reduction. Br J Dermatol 2005;152:1304–12.

32. Keystone EC, Schiff MH, Kremer JM, et al. Once-weekly administration of 50 mg etanercept in patients with active rheumatoid arthritis: results of a multicenter, randomized, double-blind, placebo-controlled trial. Arthritis Rheum 2004;50:353–63.

33. Mease PJ, Kivitz AJ, Burch FX, et al. Etanercept treatment of psoriatic arthritis: safety, efficacy, and effect on disease progression. Arthritis Rheum 2004;50:2264–72.

34. Leonardi CL, Powers JL, Matheson RT, et al, Etanercept Psoriasis Study Group. Etanercept as monotherapy in patients with psoriasis. N Engl J Med 2003;349: 2014–22.

35. Davis JC Jr, van der Heijde D, Braun J, et al, Enbrel Ankylosing Spondylitis Study Group. Recombinant human tumor necrosis factor receptor (etanercept) for treating ankylosing spondylitis: a randomized, controlled trial. Arthritis Rheum 2003; 48:3230–6.

36. Gottlieb AB, Matheson RT, Lowe N, et al. A randomized trial of etanercept as monotherapy for psoriasis. Arch Dermatol 2003;139:1627–32.

37. Bathon JM, Martin RW, Fleischmann RM, et al. A comparison of etanercept and methotrexate in patients with early rheumatoid arthritis. N Engl J Med 2000; 343:1586–93.

38. Moreland LW, Schiff MH, Baumgartner SW, et al. Etanercept therapy in rheumatoid arthritis. A randomized, controlled trial. Ann Intern Med 1999;130:478–86.

39. Westhovens R, Yocum D, Han J, et al, START Study Group. The safety of infliximab, combined with background treatments, among patients with rheumatoid arthritis and various comorbidities: a large, randomized, placebo-controlled trial. Arthritis Rheum 2006;54:1075–86.

40. Reich K, Nestle FO, Papp K, et al, EXPRESS study investigators. Infliximab induction and maintenance therapy for moderate-to-severe psoriasis: a phase III, multicentre, double-blind trial. Lancet 2005;366:1367–74.

41. Kavanaugh A, Krueger GG, Beutler A, et al, IMPACT 2 Study Group. Infliximab maintains a high degree of clinical response in patients with active psoriatic arthritis through 1 year of treatment: results from the IMPACT 2 trial. Ann Rheum Dis 2007;66:498–505.

42. Antoni CE, Kavanaugh A, Kirkham B, et al. Sustained benefits of infliximab therapy for dermatologic and articular manifestations of psoriatic arthritis: results from the infliximab multinational psoriatic arthritis controlled trial (IMPACT). Arthritis Rheum 2005;52:1227–36.

43. van der Heijde D, Dijkmans B, Geusens P, et al, Ankylosing Spondylitis Study for the Evaluation of Recombinant Infliximab Therapy Study Group. Efficacy and safety of infliximab in patients with ankylosing spondylitis: results of a randomized, placebo-controlled trial (ASSERT). Arthritis Rheum 2005;52:582–91.

44. Rutgeerts P, Sandborn WJ, Feagan BG, et al. Infliximab for induction and maintenance therapy for ulcerative colitis Act I & II. N Engl J Med 2005;353: 2462–76.

45. St Clair EW, van der Heijde DM, Smolen JS, et al. Combination of infliximab and methotrexate therapy for early rheumatoid arthritis: a randomized, controlled trial. Arthritis Rheum 2004;50:3432–43.

46. Maini R, St Clair EW, Breedveld F, et al. Infliximab (chimeric anti-tumour necrosis factor alpha monoclonal antibody) versus placebo in rheumatoid arthritis patients receiving concomitant methotrexate: a randomised phase III trial. ATTRACT Study Group. Lancet 1999;354:1932–9.

47. Present DH, Rutgeerts P, Targan S, et al. Infliximab for the treatment of fistulas in patients with Crohn's disease. N Engl J Med 1999;340:1398–405.

48. Maini RN, Breedveld FC, Kalden JR, et al. Therapeutic efficacy of multiple intravenous infusions of anti-tumor necrosis factor alpha monoclonal antibody combined with low-dose weekly methotrexate in rheumatoid arthritis. Arthritis Rheum 1998;41:1552–63.

49. Keystone EC, Ware CF. Tumor necrosis factor and anti-tumor necrosis factor therapies. J Rheumatol Suppl 2010;85:27–39.

50. Dixon WG, Kezouh A, Bernatsky S, et al. The influence of systemic glucocorticoid therapy upon the risk of non-serious infection in older patients with rheumatoid arthritis: a nested case-control study. Ann Rheum Dis 2011;70(6):956–60.

51. Strangfeld A, Listing J, Herzer P, et al. Risk of herpes zoster in patients with rheumatoid arthritis treated with anti-TNF-alpha agents. JAMA 2009;301(7): 737–44.

52. Tubach F, Salmon D, Ravaud P, et al. Risk of tuberculosis is higher with anti–tumor necrosis factor monoclonal antibody therapy than with soluble tumor necrosis factor receptor therapy: the three-year prospective French research axed on tolerance of biotherapies registry. Arthritis Rheum 2009;60(7):1884–94.

53. Wallis RS, Broder MS, Wong JY, et al. Granulomatous infectious diseases associated with tumor necrosis factor antagonists. Clin Infect Dis 2004;38(9): 1261–5.

54. Salmon-Ceron D, Tubach F, Lortholary O, et al. Drug-specific risk of nontuberculosis opportunistic infections in patients receiving anti-TNF therapy reported to the 3-year prospective French RATIO registry. Ann Rheum Dis 2011; 70(4):616–23.

55. Mitoma H, Horiuchi T, Tsukamoto H, et al. Mechanisms for cytotoxic effects of anti-tumor necrosis factor agents on transmembrane tumor necrosis factor–expressing cells: comparison among infliximab, etanercept, and adalimumab. Arthritis Rheum 2008;58:1248–57.

56. Leombruno JP, Einarson TR, Keystone EC. The safety of anti-tumour necrosis factor treatments in rheumatoid arthritis: meta and exposure-adjusted pooled analyses of serious adverse events. Ann Rheum Dis 2009;68(7):1136–45.
57. Askling J, Fored CM, Brandt L, et al. Time-dependent increase in risk of hospitalisation with infection among Swedish RA-patients treated with TNF- antagonists. Ann Rheum Dis 2007;66(10):1339–44.
58. Solomon DH, Lunt M, Schneeweiss S. The risk of infection associated with tumor necrosis factor alpha antagonists: making sense of epidemiologic evidence. Arthritis Rheum 2008;58(4):919–28.
59. Du Pan SM, Dehler S, Ciurea A, et al. Comparison of drug retention rates and causes of drug discontinuation between anti-tumor necrosis factor agents in rheumatoid arthritis. Arthritis Rheum 2009;61(5):560–8.
60. Grijalva CG, Chen L, Delzell E, et al. Initiation of tumor necrosis factor-α antagonists and the risk of hospitalization for infection in patients with autoimmune diseases. JAMA 2011;306(21):2331–9.

Infections and Biologic Therapy in Rheumatoid Arthritis
Our Changing Understanding of Risk and Prevention

Kevin L. Winthrop, MD, MPH

KEYWORDS

- Infections • Biologic therapy • Rheumatoid arthritis • Infection risk
- Infection prevention • Screening

KEY POINTS

- Patients with rheumatoid arthritis are at higher risk for serious infections and death from infection than the general public.
- Prednisone and biologic agents increase this risk, although the risk associated with biologics can be mitigated when such agents act as prednisone-sparing therapies.
- Some of the important causes of infectious morbidity in this setting are preventable with screening (eg, tuberculosis) or vaccination (eg, herpes zoster).

INCREASED INFECTIOUS RISK IN RHEUMATOID ARTHRITIS

Patients with rheumatoid arthritis (RA) have long been recognized to suffer a greater burden of serious infection. The precise immune derangements of RA that predispose to infection are not clearly known. Patients with RA seem to have reduced capacity to generate new T lymphocytes, and their T-lymphocyte repertoire becomes severely contracted over time,[1] a phenomenon perhaps akin to the immunosenescence observed in a normal aging host.[2] However, it is likely that a variety of RA-associated host factors predispose patients toward infection, including the physical derangements (eg, destruction of articular surfaces, airway inflammation) that might also impair local immunity or provide a respite for circulating pathogens. In the prebiologic era, Doran and colleagues[3] reported this heightened risk within an RA cohort study in Minnesota's Mayo Clinic patient population (**Table 1**). Compared with matched non-RA controls, the investigators documented serious infections to occur nearly twice as frequently in patients with RA, at a rate of 9/100 patients per year.

Public Health and Preventive Medicine, Oregon Health & Science University, CEI, 3375 Southwest, Terwilliger Boulevard, Portland, OR, USA
E-mail address: winthrop@ohsu.edu

Rheum Dis Clin N Am 38 (2012) 727–745
http://dx.doi.org/10.1016/j.rdc.2012.08.019
0889-857X/12/$ – see front matter © 2012 Elsevier Inc. All rights reserved.
rheumatic.theclinics.com

Table 1
The prebiologic era: frequency of infections among patients with RA and healthy controls from a Minnesota cohort

Infection Type	Incidence per 100 Patient-Years RA	Incidence per 100 Patient-Years Non-RA	Relative Risk (95% Confidence Interval)
Pneumonia	4.0	2.4	1.7 (1.5–1.9)
Skin	3.0	0.9	3.3 (2.7–4.1)
Sepsis	0.78	0.51	1.5 (1.1–2.1)
Septic joint	0.40	0.02	14.9 (6.1–73.7)
Intra-abdominal	0.22	0.08	2.8 (1.4–6.2)
Osteomyelitis	0.17	0.01	10.6 (3.4–126.8)

Data from Doran MF, Crowson CS, Pond GR, et al. Frequency of infection in patients with rheumatoid arthritis compared with controls: a population-based study. Arthritis Rheum 2002;46(9):2287–93.

This increased risk remained even after controlling for the effects of important comorbidities and other infectious risks, and similar to historical reports, these investigators documented pulmonary and skin/soft tissue infections to be the most common sites of RA-related infectious morbidity.

PREDNISONE

Although conflicting data (to be discussed later) foster debate regarding the infectious risks of biologic therapies, there is little debate regarding the ability of prednisone to cause infectious harm. Although a recent meta-analysis of glucocorticoid trials in rheumatic disease found no increased risk of serious infection associated with steroids,[4] observational studies consistently report such an association. The prebiologic era observational study of Doran and colleagues[3] documented a significant 1.5-fold to 2-fold increase in risk with corticosteroid therapy, with risk noted even at a low dose (eg, <15 mg/d) of prednisone. In 2006, Wolfe and colleagues[5] produced similar findings with increased risks (hazard ratio 1.4, 95% confidence interval [CI] 1.1–1.6) noted even at doses of prednisone less than 5 mg/d. More recent registry data further attest to the association of prednisone with serious infection. In the United States, a national collaboration of observational databases (the Safety Assessment in Biologic Therapy [SABER]) compared the risk of serious bacterial infection in patients starting biologics with methotrexate-treated patients who start an additional nonbiologic disease-modifying antirheumatic drug (DMARD). These researchers also documented dose-dependent increases in risk, with relative risk (RR) up to 3-fold higher in patients using doses greater than 10 mg/d (**Table 2**).[6] The Consortium of Rheumatology Researchers of North America (CORRONA) registry identified 1.5-fold higher risks with prednisone use for opportunistic infections, and other US studies support the idea that risk is increased even at low daily doses of 5 mg or less (1.3-fold–1.5-fold), escalating with increasing doses to 5-fold higher risk at doses of 20 mg or grerater.[7,8] Within Europe, the results have been no different. The British Society for Rheumatology Biologic Register (BSRBR), a UK cohort of patients with inflammatory arthritis, observed corticosteroids to double the risk of serious infection.[9] In Germany's biologic registry for patients with RA (RABBIT), the independent increase in relative serious infection risk observed with corticosteroids varied between 2-fold and nearly 5-fold at dosages less than 15 mg and 15 mg or greater daily, respectively.[10]

Table 2
Dose-dependent increase in hospitalized infection observed with glucocorticoid use, from the SABER study

Exposures	Events, Number	Person-Years, Number	Rate, per 100 Person-Years	Hazard Ratio (95% CI) for Propensity Score-Matched Cohorts	Adjusted Hazard Ratios (95% CI)
RA Nonbiologic regimens	326	4192	7.78	Ref.[1]	Ref.[1]
Tumor necrosis factor α antagonists	497	6089	8.16	1.05 (0.91–1.21)	1.05 (0.91–1.21)
Baseline glucocorticoid use, prednisone equivalents					
None					Ref.[1]
>0–<5 mg/d					1.32 (1.10–1.58)
5–10 mg/d					1.78 (1.47–2.15)
>10 mg/d					2.95 (2.41–3.61)

Data from Grijalva CG, Chen L, Delzell E, et al. Initiation of tumor necrosis factor-alpha antagonists and the risk of hospitalization for infection in patients with autoimmune diseases. JAMA 2011;306:2331–9.

Beyond bacterial infections, corticosteroids increase the risk of tuberculosis (TB), nontuberculous mycobacterial disease (NTM), and other opportunistic infections.[11–13] This risk has been particularly well documented with herpes zoster, in which the risk is increased 1.5 to 2 times in patients with RA who use corticosteroids.[14–16] Pulmonary NTM disease, of which patients with RA are at higher risk, has been linked to systemic prednisone and even inhaled corticosteroid use.[12–14] Disease caused by *Pneumocystis jiroveci* occurs in the setting of high-dose prednisone use, although the threshold of dose and duration of prednisone use for causing *Pneumocystis* has not been well described.[17]

Collectively, these data suggest that systemic corticosteroid use is an important and potentially modifiable risk factor for serious infection. Further, the serious infection risks observed within these studies are similar and sometimes exceed those observed with biologic therapy. Despite these infectious risks and the advent of newer biologic therapies, corticosteroid use in RA remains common.[18] Patients who use both biologic therapy and prednisone concurrently have an even higher risk of serious infection than patients who use only biologic therapy (**Fig. 1**).[10] Clearly, one of the potential benefits of DMARD therapy, either synthetic or biologic, is the opportunity to mitigate risks associated with corticosteroids by allowing for the reduction or elimination of prednisone.

Biologic Therapies

In little more than the last decade, biologic therapies targeting tumor necrosis factor α (TNF-α), T and B lymphocytes, and various interleukins (IL) (including IL-6 and IL-1) have been developed and approved for use in RA and selected other rheumatic diseases. Additional drugs with novel targets are either approved or in trials for RA and other inflammatory conditions, including those that inhibit IL-12 to IL-23 and IL-17a.

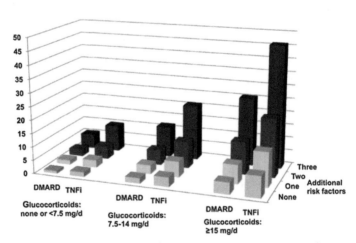

Fig. 1. Estimated incidences of serious infections in 100 patients per year by treatment and risk profile. Additional risk factors are 1 or 2 of the following: age greater than 60 years, chronic lung disease, chronic renal disease, or high number of treatment failures; 3 risk factors: 2 of these risk factors plus previous serious infections. TNFi, tumor necrosis factor inhibitor. (*From* Strangfeld A, Eveslage M, Schneider M, et al. Treatment benefit or survival of the fittest: what drives the time-dependent decrease in serious infection rates under TNF inhibition and what does this imply for the individual patient? Ann Rheum Dis 2011; 70:1914–20.)

Novel small molecules (technically not biologics) that target the janus activating kinases (JAK) and splenic tyrosine kinases are also in development, and at least one JAK inhibitor (tofacitinib) is under consideration by the US Food and Drug Administration (FDA) for approval.

Infection risk

Data from randomized controlled trials and long-term extension studies of biologic therapies have generally (but not always) suggested some increase in infectious risks associated with these compounds. For anti-TNF therapies, where abundant registry and administrative health care-based observational studies have been conducted, higher absolute infection rates among anti-TNF users have generally been observed, particularly in the 6 to 12 months after drug start. These rates observed in such real world settings have typically been higher than those observed during clinical trials and long-term extension studies. However, the assessment of infection risk with anti-TNF therapies in population-based studies is complex, and only in the last 1 to 2 years perhaps, a clearer picture has emerged. For the more recently approved biologics in RA with different mechanisms of action (ie, abatacept, tocilizumab, rituximab), rates of serious infection observed in clinical trials have largely been similar to those observed in anti-TNF trials. However, for these newer compounds, real world infection rates and risk estimates are largely missing, because such observational registry or database studies with these therapies have yet to be conducted.

Anti-TNF therapy

Five TNF blockers currently fill the marketplace: etanercept (Enbrel), infliximab (Remicade), adalimumab (Humira), golimumab (Simponi), and certolizumab (Cimzia). As a group, these drugs inhibit TNF-α, a proinflammatory cytokine expressed by activated macrophages, T lymphocytes, and other immune cells, known to play a crucial role in the host response against a variety of infections.[14] TNF directly activates macrophages to phagocytose and kill mycobacteria and a variety of other pathogens, and the failure to control TB during TNF blockade seems intrinsically linked to an inability to control intracellular TB growth in macrophages residing within granulomas,[19] rather than inhibiting the development granulomas per se.[20] Murine studies suggest the importance of TNF in protection against other intracellular organisms such as *Listeria* and fungi, as well as against extracellular bacterial organisms like *Klebsiella pneumoniae* and *Streptococcus pneumoniae*.[21–25]

Risk of infection with anti-TNF therapy

The overall risk of serious infections attributable to anti-TNF therapy is not precisely known, and our understanding of this issue depends largely on the study settings and methodology used to assess these risks. Further, much of the variability in an individual's infection risk is not attributable to drug therapy, but rather to patient factors (eg, age, chronic lung disease, and other comorbidities) that are frequently not modifiable.[8,10] Although conflicting evidence from a variety of study designs exists, it is our opinion that anti-TNF therapy independently increases the risk of serious infection, but that this risk is mitigated by a variety of measurable (and unmeasurable) factors after drug start. As suggested earlier, TNF blockers can, and should, serve as prednisone-sparing therapies, allowing for a reduction in prednisone-associated infection risk. Other physician-patient decisions such as TB screening, vaccination, counseling with regard to infection prevention, and other factors likely also serve to mitigate infectious risk associated with starting anti-TNF therapy. It is likely that patients starting anti-TNF therapies are treated differently with regard to these and other factors compared with patients starting nonbiologic DMARDs. This confounding by indication can be difficult to measure and control for in "real world" observational studies that seek to measure differences in risk between anti-TNF and nonbiologic DMARD users.

Our understanding of infection risk derives from individual randomized controlled trials and their meta-analyses, long-term open-label extension studies, and the observational (registry and database) studies, as discussed earlier. Meta-analyses of TNF-blocker trials generally observed RRs of serious infection to be slightly higher in those patients treated with anti-TNF therapy, but not always so, and frequently the observed effect has been mild and not statistically significant. Bongartz and colleagues[26] analyzed monoclonal antibody trials (infliximab and adalimumab only) in RA and observed a 2-fold increase in serious infection risk. Leombruno and colleagues[27] evaluated serious infection risk within RA trials of etanercept, infliximab, and adalimumab and found no statistically increased risk (RR 1.08 [0.81–1.43]) in those treated with anti-TNF therapy versus placebo overall, but did find a significant 2-fold increase in risk for those studies using higher-dose infliximab or adalimumab. More recently, Singh and colleagues[28] preformed a Cochrane review of anti-TNF therapies across disease indications and found infliximab (odds ratio [OR] 1.45 [0.99–2.1]) and certolizumab (OR 3.5 [1.6–7.8]) to have the highest RR of serious infection compared with placebo, whereas no other TNF blockers were shown to have significant increased risk. There are great difficulties in understanding the infectious profiles relying on data from randomized controlled trials (eg, statistical power is low for individual trials, careful selection of patients), and even greater difficulties in comparing drugs across trials (eg, differences in inclusion criteria, populations, disease indications, others), such that it is unclear from such meta-analytical studies if drugs like infliximab or certolizumab carry any greater risk than other TNF blockers.

Lastly, it is worth noting that trials involving patients with ages and conditions associated with lower baseline infectious risk, such as psoriasis, have observed lower overall rates and relative risks of serious infection in patients using these therapies.[29–31]

Several large observational studies and registries have also assessed the risk of infection with these compounds. Although these studies have heterogeneity in methods and cannot fully overcome issues of confounding (eg, confounding by indication), these studies have reported similar estimates of serious infection in patients using these therapies. The incidence of serious infection for patients with RA using TNF blockers generally hovers between 3 and 8/100 patient-years (**Table 3**), and both absolute and relative rates seem dependent on when they are measured after drug start.[8,32,33] The BSRBR found a 4-fold increase in risk for serious infection in the first 90 days after anti-TNF start among patients with RA, and Curtis and colleagues[8] reported a similar increased risk in the first 6 months after anti-TNF start.[34] Both studies produced smaller RR estimates when longer periods of exposure were assessed. This finding is likely because of a survivor effect, but also potentially secondary to benefits of improved disease management, and changes in concomitant therapies, which occur after anti-TNF therapy start.[10]

Grijalva and colleagues[35] recently published results from the SABER collaboration, a population-based study that compared only new users in both groups: anti-TNF or nonbiologic DMARDs. Within RA, this comparison was restricted to those patients failing methotrexate who subsequently started either an anti-TNF drug (for the first time) or a new nonbiologic DMARD. Although the influence of baseline corticosteroid use, comorbidities, and disease severity was controlled for in modeling, changes taking place after drug start (eg, changes in prednisone, concomitant nonbiologic DMARD use, improved disease control) could not be assessed. Although investigators reported high rates of serious infection (8/100 patient-years for RA), no increased risk

Table 3
The biologic era: rates and RRs of serious infections in patients with RA using anti-TNF therapy from European and North American observational cohort studies

Country, Year	Crude Incidence per 100 Patient-Years Anti-TNF Treated	Crude Incidence per 100 Patient-Years Nonbiologic Comparator	Adjusted RR[a] (95% CI)
Germany,[37] 2005	6.4, ETN 6.2, INF	2.3	2.2 (0.9–5.4) ETN 2.1 (0.8–5.5) INF
United Kingdom,[34] 2007	5.5	3.9	1.3 (0.9–1.8)[c] 4.6 (1.8–11.9)[b]
United States,[8] 2007	2.9[d]	1.4[d]	4.2 (2.0–8.8)[d] 1.9 (1.3–2.8)
Sweden,[32] 2007	4.7	NR	1.4 (1.2–1.7)[e]
United States,[7] 2007	4.9	3.8	1.3 (0.8–2.1)
United States,[35] 2011	8.2	7.8	1.05 (0.9–1.2)
Germany,[10] 2011	4.8	2.3	1.8 (1.2–2.7)[f]
Japan,[91] 2011	6.4	2.6	2.4 (1.1–5.05)[g]

Abbreviations: ETN, etanercept; INF, infliximab; NR, not reported.
  [a] Relative rate using nonbiologic users as the referent.
  [b] When restricted to the first 90 days of therapy, and adjusted for age, sex, disease duration, and severity, extra-articular RA, baseline steroid use, diabetes, chronic obstructive pulmonary disease, pulmonary disease, and smoking history.
  [c] Adjusted relative rate when not restricted to the first 90 days of therapy.
  [d] Analysis restricted to the first 6 months after initiation of anti-TNF therapy.
  [e] Rate calculated at 1 year after starting treatment and adjusted for RA severity and comorbidities associated with infections.
  [f] Adjustment for time-varying risk factors, treatment adaptations, and dropout.
  [g] Rate up to 1 year after drug start.

was associated with anti-TNF therapy start (see **Table 2**) and contrary to the previous observational studies discussed earlier, no short-term increased risk was noted in the first 3 to 6 months after drug start. Within their RA cohort, these investigators found that infliximab starters were 20% to 25% more likely to suffer serious infection than those who started with either etanercept or adalimumab. However, patients starting infliximab were more likely to be on methotrexate after the index date than those starting etanercept or adalimumab, perhaps contributing to this increase in risk. Other population-based studies have failed to find a similar increase in RR for bacterial infections with infliximab compared with the other TNF blockers.[33,36,37] The study reiterated the importance of patient factors to overall infection risk. For example, patients treated with anti-TNF with a history of chronic obstructive pulmonary disease (COPD) had rates of nearly 17 versus 7 per 100 patient-years for those without COPD.

Collectively, the observational studies conducted to date suggest that the overall or net infectious risk of biologic therapy is not straightforward to understand or calculate, and that one must account for time-varying risk factors during such study. Strangfeld and colleagues[10] examined this issue using the RABBIT registry and were able to control for several factors that either increase or decrease the risk of infection after drug start. Their data suggest that anti-TNF therapy start improves disease control and decreases prednisone use, both lowering infectious risk, but that even when controlling for these changes, the start of anti-TNF therapy significantly increases the risk of serious infections 1.8-fold. This study arguably represents our most complete understanding of the dynamic risk profile presented by these therapies. We know less regarding serious infectious risks of the 2 newer anti-TNF therapies certolizumab and golimumab, because large population-based studies of these compounds are lacking.

Opportunistic infections with anti-TNF therapy

Several intracellular and other opportunistic pathogens have been reported in the setting of anti-TNF therapy (**Tables 4** and **5**). These pathogens include severe and sometimes lethal infections with *Histoplasma, Coccidioides, Listeria, Salmonella, Aspergillus, Nocardia*, and nontuberculous mycobacteria.[38] Of these infections, TB is most clearly associated with TNF blockade, and a clear distinction in risk can be made between the fusion receptor construct etanercept, and that of the monoclonal antibodies infliximab and adalimumab. Although TB risk has been documented to be clearly increased with all 3 drugs, it is 3-fold to 4-fold more common in adalimumab-treated and infliximab-treated patients relative to etanercept.[39,40] Several animal and in vitro studies support the biological plausibility of these observations. Potential explanations range from differential granuloma penetration to differential downregulation of antigen-stimulated interferon-γ to differential affects on antimicrobial-producing CD8 effector cells.[41–43] Cases of TB have been reported from clinical trial experience of certolizumab and golimumab, but few population data exist by which to compare their RR with the other TNF blockers.

The incidence of TB and RR of anti-TNF therapy directly reflects the a priori risk of the exposed population. Early population-based studies from regions of low TB prevalence generally reported rates of TB 5 to 20 times higher than background populations, including early studies from the United States (incidence of 52/100,000) and Sweden (incidence of 118/100,000) largely before the widespread introduction of mandatory screening for TB before biologic initiation.[44,45] Spanish investigators reported estimated rates of 1900/100,000, approximately 10-fold to 20-fold higher among RA anti-TNF users compared with biologic-naive patients with RA. These rates have since decreased dramatically with institution of widespread screening for latent TB infection before anti-TNF use.[46] More recently, formal observational studies conducted within France, the United Kingdom, and the United States have documented rates of between 56 and 117/100,000 (see **Table 5**). Work in the United States suggests that disease caused by nontuberculous mycobacteria occurs approximately

Table 4
The biologic era: rates and RRs of opportunistic infections in patients with RA using anti-TNF therapy from European and North American observational cohort studies

Country, Year	Outcome Studied	Crude Incidence per 100,000 Patient-Years Anti-TNF Treated	Crude Incidence per 100,000 Patient-Years Nonbiologic Comparator	Adjusted RR[b] (95% CI)
United Kingdom,[33] 2006	OI	192[b,c]	0[b]	NR
France,[92] 2006	OI[d]	152[a]	NR	NR
United States,[93] 2010	OI	3000[b]	1600[b]	1.7 (0.95–2.9)

Abbreviations: NR, not reported; UNDEF, undefined.
 [a] Rate adjusted for age and sex.
 [b] Cohorts restricted to patients with RA.
 [c] Rate not published, but was estimated using data provided within the article.
 [d] OI outcomes did not include TB.

Table 5
The biologic era: rates and RRs of specific opportunistic infections in patients with RA using anti-TNF therapy from European and North American observational cohort studies

Country, Year	Outcome Studied	Crude Incidence per 100,000 Patient-Years Anti-TNF Treated	Crude Incidence per 100,000 Patient-Years Nonbiologic Comparator	Adjusted RR[b] (95% CI)
United Kingdom,[39] 2010	TB	95[b]	0[b]	UNDEF
France,[92] 2011	TB	117[a]	NR	NR
United States,[94] 2011	TB	56[b]	9[b]	NR
United States,[82] 2011	NTM	105[b]	19[b]	NR
France,[92] 2006	Legionella pneumonia	37.5[c]	NR	NR
United States,[95] 2009	Zoster	1060	1118	NR
Germany,[10] 2011	Zoster	980[b]	560[b]	1.63
United Kingdom,[36] 2011	Zoster	1600	800	1.7

Abbreviations: NR, not reported; NTM, nontuberculous; TB, tuberculosis; UNDEF, undefined.
[a] Rate adjusted for age and sex.
[b] Cohorts restricted to patients with RA.
[c] Average of estimated rate.

twice more frequently than TB in the anti-TNF setting, perhaps not surprising given the low background TB prevalence in the country.[40,47] In the context of biologic therapy, pulmonary NTM disease is associated with RA, because these environmental organisms (most commonly *Mycobacterium avium* complex) have a predilection for patients with underlying lung disease.[40] Like TB, extrapulmonary manifestations of NTM disease seem to be more common among patients using anti-TNF therapies.[48]

For other intracellular and opportunistic infections, there remain fewer data by which to estimate risk. Several studies have looked at opportunistic infections, although risk estimates vary wildly between studies because study methods and case definitions for opportunistic infections frequently differ (see **Table 4**). The CORRONA database documented rates of opportunistic infections 20 times higher than the French study, but CORRONA consider all cases of herpes zoster within their outcome where the French study considered only multidermatomal zoster cases.

Zoster is the most common opportunistic infection in this setting, and occurs more frequently in patients with RA. Its risk is clearly increased by the use of prednisone, but data regarding the risk of anti-TNF therapy are conflicting.[14] Although investigators from RABBIT and BSRBR have documented increased risks with anti-TNF therapy, 1 large study within the US Veterans Affairs found no increased risk with anti-TNF therapy (see **Table 5**). Further, whereas the RABBIT registry suggested that zoster occurred significantly more frequently in those treated with adalimumab and infliximab compared with etanercept, the BSRBR data suggested adalimumab to be protective relative to etanercept. Other organism-specific data exist for *Legionella* (from France) in which TNF antagonist users were at higher risk. Although there are great disparities in rates, risk estimates, and study methodologies, the overall picture is that anti-TNF therapy does increase the risk of many infections considered opportunistic, in particular those that involve granulomatous host response. Like for TB, the risk of many other opportunistic infections such as the endemic mycoses (histoplasmosis, coccidoidomycosis, blastomycosis) vary according to geography and baseline risk.

THE OTHER BIOLOGICS: ABATACEPT, RITUXIMAB, TOCILIZUMAB, AND ANAKINRA

Primarily reserved for those patients who have failed or have contraindications for anti-TNF therapy, these newer biologics are important additions to the RA therapeutic armamentarium. rituximab (Rituxin), approved for RA in 2006, is an anti-CD20 B-lymphocyte depletion agent; abatacept (Orencia), a CTLA-4 ligand, blocks CD80/86 interactions on CD4 T lymphocytes and mitigates their activation; and tocilizumab (Actemra) blocks the IL-6 receptor. Given these mechanisms of action, a variety of related infections are possible, and similar infection profiles have emerged with these agents to those with anti-TNF agents, although with some notable exceptions and a caveat that postmarketing experience and observational data are young with these compounds.

Risk of Serious Infections, Including Opportunistic Infections

Clinical trials with rituximab among patients with RA did not suggest a significantly increased risk of serious infection.[49] Long-term extension studies and meta-analyses data suggest that small subgroups of treated patients develop persistent hypogammaglobulinemia and are at increased risk of serious infection.[50,51] One observational study examined hospitalized infection rates among patients switching biologics, and found that those switching to rituximab had a similar risk to those switching to etanercept, adalimumab, and abatacept (and significantly lower risk than those who switched to infliximab).[52] There are case reports of both TB and NTM disease in patients on rituximab, although these patients have also been on methotrexate and prednisone.[47,53] Rituximab use in patients with chronic hepatitis B virus (HBV) is contraindicated, and treated patients (primarily reported from the lymphoma setting) have suffered HBV reactivation and death.[28,54,55] In addition, rare cases of progressive multifocal leukoencephalopathy (PML) have been reported in patients with RA using rituximab and more rarely anti-TNF therapies. In general, PML is rare outside the setting of human immunodeficiency virus (incidence in RA estimated at 1/1,000,000)[56] and the risk is unknown in those using rituximab or other biologic therapies. At least 14 cases of PML occurring in rituximab-treated patients with inflammatory diseases have been reported to the FDA, although 10 were using other immunosuppressive therapies in addition to rituximab and only 1 patient lacked any other identifiable potential risk factors for PML.[57]

For abatacept, some clinical trials suggested a small increased risk of serious infection, particularly respiratory infections and exacerbations in those with COPD.[58,59] The risk of serious infections was significantly increased when abatacept was combined with anti-TNF therapy.[59–61] Subsequent meta-analyses of randomized controlled trial data suggested a nonsignificant trend toward an increase in serious infection compared with placebo,[49] and similar analyses that included open-label extension data documented rates of hospitalized infection of 2.7/100 patient-years for patients using abatacept.[62] For TB and other opportunistic infections, cases have been reported, although the RR of these types of infections is not yet known. The rate of observed TB in the double-blind portion of abatacept RA trials was 60/100,000 patient-years.[62] In animal studies, abatacept does not seem to negatively affect the immune system of mice that are exposed to TB.[63] In humans, Schiff and colleagues[64] recently conducted a randomized trial to compare the efficacy and safety of abatacept with infliximab. At 12 months of follow-up, patients using abatacept suffered significantly fewer serious infections than infliximab-treated patients (1.9% vs 8.5%), with a rate similar to that seen in the placebo group at 6 months' follow-up (2.7%). No cases of opportunistic infections were seen in the abatacept-treated group, although 5 such cases were seen in the infliximab group, including 2 cases of TB and 1 case of *Pneumocystis jiroveci* pneumonia.

For tocilizumab, the rates and types of serious infection from randomized controlled and long-term extension trials were generally similar to those from other biologic trials. Serious infection rates were 4.9 per 100 patient-years in patients using 8 mg/kg dosing, whereas rates (3.5/100 patient-years) were observed in those receiving placebo or low-dose tocilizumab.[65] Postmarketing population-based observational data are limited, although a group in Japan recently published from their tocilizumab postmarketing surveillance program, which included 3881 treated patients. Serious infection rates of 9/100 patient-years were observed, and rates of herpes zoster were 6.1/1000 patient-years.[66] In addition, 4 cases of TB were recorded (incidence rate 220/100,000), a rate approximately 10-fold higher than the background Japanese population, but a rate similar to that observed in the postmarketing experience for anti-TNF therapies in Japan.

ANAKINRA

This recombinant IL-1 receptor antagonist is used infrequently within RA. It has been shown to significantly increase the risk of serious infection, particularly when combined with prednisone or anti-TNF therapy.[67,68] Clear warnings exist that concurrent anti-TNF therapy with anakinra should be avoided.[68]

TOFACITINIB

Few data have been published regarding the infectious risks of tofacitinib, a novel small molecule that inhibits JAK 1/3 and is technically not a biologic, data from a large international clinical development program in RA were recently presented to the FDA and a decision regarding licensure is pending. In vitro, this drug has been shown to diminish CD4 T-lymphocyte production of INF-γ and IL-17.[69] Infections such as TB, herpes zoster, or others that are dependent on host INF-γ responses could be expected given this mechanism of action, and some cases of opportunistic infections have been reported in abstract form.[70] Only several small phase II studies from the RA program have been published in the peer-reviewed literature. In these small trials, patients receiving 5-mg and 10-mg twice daily doses had serious infection rates, similar to that in placebo groups, although neutropenia did occur more frequently with tofacitinib.[71,72]

Prevention of Infection in Patients Using Biologics (Screening and Vaccination)

It is likely that the serious bacterial infections most common in this setting, such as community-acquired pneumonia and skin/soft tissue infections, are caused by the same types of organisms seen in the general public.[5,37,73] Most skin/soft tissue infections are likely caused by *Staphylococcus aureus* and *Streptococcus* sp,[74] although few organism-level incidence data have been published in this setting. It is unclear whether such infections can be prevented, and it is unclear whether colonization with *Staphylococcus aureus* is a risk for subsequent infection in patients who go on to biologic therapy. Many patients with RA are also hospitalized each year with community-acquired pneumonia, and these infections too are likely caused by the same organisms that cause pneumonia in general populations: *Streptococcus pneumoniae, Haemophilus influenza, Staphylococcus aureus*, gram-negative bacilli, and influenza are some of the most common causes.[75] For *Streptococcus pneumoniae*, patients are recommended to receive 23-valent pneumococcal vaccine before initiating anti-TNF and other long-term immunosuppressive therapies (primarily for protection against invasive pneumococcal disease).[76] Immunogenicity to this vaccine is poor and diminished by methotrexate as well as some other biologic drugs (eg, rituximab), but is relatively unaffected by anti-TNF therapy.[77] Recently, the FDA has approved the new 13-valent conjugate pneumococcal vaccine (PCV13) for use in adults. This vaccine theoretically provides longer and improved protection against pneumococcal disease.[78] The American College of Immunization Practices recently voted to recommend PCV13 in patients with certain immunocompromising conditions, although their formal and official recommendation with regard to its use (particularly in those formerly vaccinated with pneumovax) is still pending publication.[79]

Opportunistic and viral infections

An influenza vaccination should be given yearly and is efficacious when given during biologic therapy (although less efficacious during rituximab treatment)[80,81] It is unclear whether higher-dose influenza vaccines provide improved protection in such patients. Either usual-dose or higher-dose products are recommended until further data are available. However, the use of live intranasal influenza vaccine is contraindicated in patients using anti-TNF and other biologic therapies.

In many areas of the world, chronic hepatitis B and C are prevalent; the epidemiology of HBV closely mirrors that of TB, with similar regions of endemnicity throughout the globe.[82] Although the anti-TNF compounds seem relatively safe in patients with hepatitis C virus, HBV progression can occur in patients using anti-TNF therapy, and patients should be screened for HBV before using such therapies. Optimal screening algorithms should include evaluation of hepatitis B serum antigen, core antibody, and surface antibody, and it should include pretreatment HBV DNA evaluation in anyone with evidence of previous infection (ie, hepatitis B core antibody).[82] HBV progression and poor outcomes have been reported in patients using rituximab, although primarily from the lymphoproliferative disease setting. Data for the other non-TNF blocking biologics are scarce given their more recent introduction. Only 1 case of HBV progression has been reported in a patient using abatacept, and several patients with HBV have successfully used tocilizumab in the context of antiviral prophylaxis.[83] Although rituximab should be contraindicated in patients with active HBV, the other biologics have been successfully used in the context of concomitant antiviral therapy and close laboratory/clinical monitoring.

The reactivation of varicella virus (ie, herpes zoster) remains a potentially preventable disease for patients with RA using biologic therapy. Regardless of whether biologic therapy increases the risk of herpes zoster, it is clear that patients with RA as they age are at increasing risk of this often debilitating disease. Zostavax is licensed for patients older than 50 years for the prevention of shingles and has been shown to reduce overall zoster risk by 67% in those vaccinated.[84] This live vaccine is contraindicated during biologic therapy, although a recent observational study suggested that patients inadvertently vaccinated while receiving anti-TNF therapy were not harmed.[85] Given the high morbidity and prevalence of this disease in RA and the inability to vaccinate patients with RA using biologic therapies, efforts should be made to evaluate the safety and efficacy of this vaccine in this context.

Of the other opportunistic infections, it is primarily TB that is truly preventable in the setting of biologic therapy. Recommendations for TB screening have been issued by various public health authorities and professional societies.[28,86,87] Interferon-γ release assays (IGRAs), QuantiFERON-TB Gold In-Tube (Cellestis, Valencia, CA), or the T-SPOT.*TB* assay (Oxford Immunotec, Abingdon, UK), which measure lymphocyte interferon-γ response to antigens highly specific to TB, are becoming increasingly used in this setting. Given the improved specificity of these tests in patients with a history of bacille Calmette-Guérin (BCG), they are preferentially recommended in regions where BCG is used. However, data suggest that screening with IGRAs or tuberculin skin test alone does not sufficiently identify all patients at risk, as false negative results can occur particularly in immunosuppressed individuals.[88] A dual testing strategy of both tuberculin skin test and IGRA (or in the case of a BCG-vaccinated individual, a dual IGRA strategy) is likely warranted, particularly in patients with risk factors for TB. Patients diagnosed with latent TB should start prophylactic antibiotic therapy before beginning their biologic.

For nontuberculous mycobacteria and fungal disease, there are few preventive tools for the clinician to use. Patients with RA are at increased risk for pulmonary NTM, and presumably some of these patients are identified during TB screening.[40,89] Screening for NTM disease before anti-TNF treatment is largely theoretical, but could be considered in any patients with abnormalities on their baseline radiograph or in those with unexplained chronic cough. Such workup could include chest computed tomography and culture of respiratory specimens.[90] Whether it is safe to pursue anti-TNF or other biologic therapy in patients with active NTM disease, treated or untreated, is unknown. For the endemic mycosis such as *Histoplasma capsulatum* and *Coccidioides immitis* and *posadasii*, the usefulness of serologic or other screening has not been established and is difficult to conceptualize in this setting. For other intracellular pathogens such as *Listeria* or *Salmonella* that are foodborne, avoidance of certain foods (uncooked meats, unpasteurized milk products), thorough cooking of meat, and washing of produce can help to prevent disease.

SUMMARY

Patients with RA are at higher risk for serious infections and death from infection than the general public. Prednisone and biologic agents increase this risk, although risk can be mitigated when such agents act as prednisone-sparing therapies. Some of the important causes of infectious morbidity in this setting are preventable with screening (ie, TB) or vaccination (ie, herpes zoster). As newer biologic, targeted therapies are developed, new infectious challenges will arise, with established and emerging pathogens. Population-based observational studies should be conducted to further elucidate the risk of the newer biologics in the marketplace, and will be of continued importance as additional agents with novel mechanisms become part of the rheumatologist's armamentarium.

ACKNOWLEDGMENTS

I thank Jennifer Ku for providing support with the literature search and formatting of this article.

REFERENCES

1. Wagner UG, Koetz K, Weyand CM, et al. Perturbation of the T cell repertoire in rheumatoid arthritis. Proc Natl Acad Sci U S A 1998;95(24):14447–52.

2. Vallejo AN, Weyand CM, Goronzy JJ. T-cell senescence: a culprit of immune abnormalities in chronic inflammation and persistent infection. Trends Mol Med 2004;10(3):119–24.
3. Doran MF, Crowson CS, Pond GR, et al. Frequency of infection in patients with rheumatoid arthritis compared with controls: a population-based study. Arthritis Rheum 2002;46(9):2287–93.
4. Dixon WG, Kezouh A, Bernatsky S, et al. The influence of systemic glucocorticoid therapy upon the risk of non-serious infection in older patients with rheumatoid arthritis: a nested case-control study. Ann Rheum Dis 2011;70(6):956–60.
5. Wolfe F, Caplan L, Michaud K. Treatment for rheumatoid arthritis and the risk of hospitalization for pneumonia: associations with prednisone, disease-modifying antirheumatic drugs, and anti-tumor necrosis factor therapy. Arthritis Rheum 2006;54(2):628–34.
6. Grijalva CG, Kaltenbach L, Arbogast PG, et al. Initiation of rheumatoid arthritis treatments and the risk of serious infections. Rheumatology (Oxford) 2010; 49(1):82–90.
7. Schneeweiss S, Setoguchi S, Weinblatt ME, et al. Anti-tumor necrosis factor alpha therapy and the risk of serious bacterial infections in elderly patients with rheumatoid arthritis. Arthritis Rheum 2007;56(6):1754–64.
8. Curtis JR, Patkar N, Xie A, et al. Risk of serious bacterial infections among rheumatoid arthritis patients exposed to tumor necrosis factor alpha antagonists. Arthritis Rheum 2007;56(4):1125–33.
9. Franklin J, Lunt M, Bunn D, et al. Risk and predictors of infection leading to hospitalisation in a large primary-care-derived cohort of patients with inflammatory polyarthritis. Ann Rheum Dis 2007;66(3):308–12.
10. Strangfeld A, Eveslage M, Schneider M, et al. Treatment benefit or survival of the fittest: what drives the time-dependent decrease in serious infection rates under TNF inhibition and what does this imply for the individual patient? Ann Rheum Dis 2011;70(11):1914–20.
11. Jick SS, Lieberman ES, Rahman MU, et al. Glucocorticoid use, other associated factors, and the risk of tuberculosis. Arthritis Rheum 2006;55(1):19–26.
12. Dirac MA, Horan KL, Doody DR, et al. Environment or host?: a case-control study of risk factors for *Mycobacterium avium* complex lung disease. Am J Respir Crit Care Med 2012. [Epub ahead of print].
13. Hojo M, Iikura M, Hirano S, et al. Increased risk of nontuberculous mycobacterial infection in asthmatic patients using long-term inhaled corticosteroid therapy. Respirology 2012;17(1):185–90.
14. Winthrop KL, Furst DE. Rheumatoid arthritis and herpes zoster: risk and prevention in those treated with anti-tumour necrosis factor therapy. Ann Rheum Dis 2010;69(10):1735–7.
15. Smitten AL, Choi HK, Hochberg MC, et al. The risk of hospitalized infection in patients with rheumatoid arthritis. J Rheumatol 2008;35(3):387–93.
16. Strangfeld A, Listing J, Herzer P, et al. Risk of herpes zoster in patients with rheumatoid arthritis treated with anti-TNF-alpha agents. JAMA 2009;301(7):737–44.
17. Yale SH, Limper AH. *Pneumocystis carinii* pneumonia in patients without acquired immunodeficiency syndrome: associated illness and prior corticosteroid therapy. Mayo Clin Proc 1996;71(1):5–13.
18. Hyrich K, Symmons D, Watson K, et al. BSRBR Control Centre Consortium, British Society for Rheumatology Biologics Register. Baseline comorbidity levels in biologic and standard DMARD treated patients with rheumatoid arthritis: results from a national patient register. Ann Rheum Dis 2006;65(7):895–8.

19. Clay H, Volkman HE, Ramakrishnan L. Tumor necrosis factor signaling mediates resistance to mycobacteria by inhibiting bacterial growth and macrophage death. Immunity 2008;29(2):283–94.
20. Lin YC, Yeh CJ, Wang LH, et al. The effect of CCND1 +870A>G and VEGF +936C>T polymorphisms on oral cancer development and disease-free survival in a Taiwan population. Oral Oncol 2012;48(6):535–40.
21. Rothe J, Lesslauer W, Lotscher H, et al. Mice lacking the tumour necrosis factor receptor 1 are resistant to TNF-mediated toxicity but highly susceptible to infection by *Listeria monocytogenes*. Nature 1993;364(6440):798–802.
22. Deepe GS Jr. Modulation of infection with *Histoplasma capsulatum* by inhibition of tumor necrosis factor-alpha activity. Clin Infect Dis 2005;41(Suppl 3):S204–7.
23. O'Brien DP, Briles DE, Szalai AJ, et al. Tumor necrosis factor alpha receptor I is important for survival from *Streptococcus pneumoniae* infections. Infect Immun 1999;67(2):595–601.
24. Moore TA, Lau HY, Cogen AL, et al. Defective innate antibacterial host responses during murine *Klebsiella pneumoniae* bacteremia: tumor necrosis factor (TNF) receptor 1 deficiency versus therapy with anti-TNF-alpha. Clin Infect Dis 2005; 41(Suppl 3):S213–7.
25. Bekker LG, Freeman S, Murray PJ, et al. TNF-alpha controls intracellular mycobacterial growth by both inducible nitric oxide synthase-dependent and inducible nitric oxide synthase-independent pathways. J Immunol 2001;166(11):6728–34.
26. Bongartz T, Sutton AJ, Sweeting MJ, et al. Anti-TNF antibody therapy in rheumatoid arthritis and the risk of serious infections and malignancies: systematic review and meta-analysis of rare harmful effects in randomized controlled trials. JAMA 2006;295(19):2275–85.
27. Leombruno JP, Einarson TR, Keystone EC. The safety of anti-tumour necrosis factor treatments in rheumatoid arthritis: meta and exposure-adjusted pooled analyses of serious adverse events. Ann Rheum Dis 2009;68(7):1136–45.
28. Singh JA, Furst DE, Bharat A, et al. 2012 update of the 2008 American College of Rheumatology recommendations for the use of disease-modifying antirheumatic drugs and biologic agents in the treatment of rheumatoid arthritis. Arthritis Care Res (Hoboken) 2012;64(5):625–39.
29. Burmester GR, Mease P, Dijkmans BA, et al. Adalimumab safety and mortality rates from global clinical trials of six immune-mediated inflammatory diseases. Ann Rheum Dis 2009;68(12):1863–9.
30. Dommasch ED, Abuabara K, Shin DB, et al. The risk of infection and malignancy with tumor necrosis factor antagonists in adults with psoriatic disease: a systematic review and meta-analysis of randomized controlled trials. J Am Acad Dermatol 2011;64(6):1035–50.
31. Pariser DM, Leonardi CL, Gordon K, et al. Integrated safety analysis: short- and long-term safety profiles of etanercept in patients with psoriasis. J Am Acad Dermatol 2012;67(2):245–56.
32. Askling J, Fored CM, Brandt L, et al. Time-dependent increase in risk of hospitalisation with infection among Swedish RA patients treated with TNF antagonists. Ann Rheum Dis 2007;66(10):1339–44.
33. Dixon WG, Watson K, Lunt M, et al. Rates of serious infection, including site-specific and bacterial intracellular infection, in rheumatoid arthritis patients receiving anti-tumor necrosis factor therapy: results from the British Society for Rheumatology Biologics Register. Arthritis Rheum 2006;54(8):2368–76.
34. Dixon WG, Symmons DP, Lunt M, et al. Serious infection following anti-tumor necrosis factor alpha therapy in patients with rheumatoid arthritis: lessons from

interpreting data from observational studies. Arthritis Rheum 2007;56(9): 2896–904.

35. Grijalva CG, Chen L, Delzell E, et al. Initiation of tumor necrosis factor-alpha antagonists and the risk of hospitalization for infection in patients with autoimmune diseases. JAMA 2011;306(21):2331–9.

36. Galloway JB, Hyrich KL, Mercer LK, et al. Risk of septic arthritis in patients with rheumatoid arthritis and the effect of anti-TNF therapy: results from the British Society for Rheumatology Biologics Register. Ann Rheum Dis 2011;70(10): 1810–4.

37. Listing J, Strangfeld A, Kary S, et al. Infections in patients with rheumatoid arthritis treated with biologic agents. Arthritis Rheum 2005;52(11):3403–12.

38. Wallis RS, Broder MS, Wong JY, et al. Granulomatous infectious diseases associated with tumor necrosis factor antagonists. Clin Infect Dis 2004;38(9):1261–5.

39. Dixon WG, Hyrich KL, Watson KD, et al. Drug-specific risk of tuberculosis in patients with rheumatoid arthritis treated with anti-TNF therapy: results from the British Society for Rheumatology Biologics Register (BSRBR). Ann Rheum Dis 2010;69(3):522–8.

40. Winthrop K, Baxter R, Liu L, et al. Mycobacterial diseases and antitumour necrosis factor therapy in USA. Ann Rheum Dis 2012. [Epub ahead of print].

41. Saliu OY, Sofer C, Stein DS, et al. Tumor-necrosis-factor blockers: differential effects on mycobacterial immunity. J Infect Dis 2006;194(4):486–92.

42. Bruns H, Meinken C, Schauenberg P, et al. Anti-TNF immunotherapy reduces CD8 + T cell-mediated antimicrobial activity against *Mycobacterium tuberculosis* in humans. J Clin Invest 2009;119(5):1167–77.

43. Plessner HL, Lin PL, Kohno T, et al. Neutralization of tumor necrosis factor (TNF) by antibody but not TNF receptor fusion molecule exacerbates chronic murine tuberculosis. J Infect Dis 2007;195(11):1643–50.

44. Askling J, Fored CM, Brandt L, et al. Risk and case characteristics of tuberculosis in rheumatoid arthritis associated with tumor necrosis factor antagonists in Sweden. Arthritis Rheum 2005;52(7):1986–92.

45. Wolfe F, Michaud K, Anderson J, et al. Tuberculosis infection in patients with rheumatoid arthritis and the effect of infliximab therapy. Arthritis Rheum 2004;50(2): 372–9.

46. Carmona L, Gomez-Reino JJ, Rodriguez-Valverde V, et al. Effectiveness of recommendations to prevent reactivation of latent tuberculosis infection in patients treated with tumor necrosis factor antagonists. Arthritis Rheum 2005; 52(6):1766–72.

47. Winthrop KL, Yamashita S, Beekmann SE, et al. Infectious Diseases Society of America Emerging Infections Network. Mycobacterial and other serious infections in patients receiving anti-tumor necrosis factor and other newly approved biologic therapies: case finding through the emerging infections network. Clin Infect Dis 2008;46(11):1738–40.

48. Winthrop KL, Chang E, Yamashita S, et al. Nontuberculous mycobacteria infections and anti-tumor necrosis factor-alpha therapy. Emerg Infect Dis 2009; 15(10):1556–61.

49. Salliot C, Dougados M, Gossec L. Risk of serious infections during rituximab, abatacept and anakinra treatments for rheumatoid arthritis: meta-analyses of randomised placebo-controlled trials. Ann Rheum Dis 2009;68(1):25–32.

50. Gottenberg JE, Ravaud P, Bardin T, et al. Risk factors for severe infections in patients with rheumatoid arthritis treated with rituximab in the autoimmunity and rituximab registry. Arthritis Rheum 2010;62(9):2625–32.

51. Furst DE, Keystone EC, Braun J, et al. Updated consensus statement on biological agents for the treatment of rheumatic diseases, 2010. Ann Rheum Dis 2011; 70(Suppl 1):i2–36.

52. Curtis JR, Xie F, Chen L, et al. The comparative risk of serious infections among rheumatoid arthritis patients starting or switching biological agents. Ann Rheum Dis 2011;70(8):1401–6.

53. Lutt JR, Pisculli ML, Weinblatt ME, et al. Severe nontuberculous mycobacterial infection in 2 patients receiving rituximab for refractory myositis. J Rheumatol 2008;35(8):1683–5.

54. Tsutsumi Y, Ogasawara R, Kamihara Y, et al. Rituximab administration and reactivation of HBV. Hepat Res Treat 2010;2010:182067.

55. Singh JA, Wells GA, Christensen R, et al. Adverse effects of biologics: a network meta-analysis and Cochrane overview. Cochrane Database Syst Rev 2011;(2):CD008794.

56. Bharat A, Xie F, Baddley JW, et al. Incidence and risk factors for progressive multifocal leukoencephalopathy among patients with selected rheumatic diseases. Arthritis Care Res (Hoboken) 2012;64(4):612–5.

57. Molloy ES, Calabrese LH. Progressive multifocal leukoencephalopathy associated with immunosuppressive therapy in rheumatic diseases: evolving role of biologic therapies. Arthritis Rheum 2012;64(9):3043–51.

58. Furst DE. The risk of infections with biologic therapies for rheumatoid arthritis. Semin Arthritis Rheum 2010;39(5):327–46.

59. Rozelle AL, Genovese MC. Efficacy results from pivotal clinical trials with abatacept. Clin Exp Rheumatol 2007;25(5 Suppl 46):S30–4.

60. Kremer JM, Genant HK, Moreland LW, et al. Effects of abatacept in patients with methotrexate-resistant active rheumatoid arthritis: a randomized trial. Ann Intern Med 2006;144(12):865–76.

61. Weinblatt M, Schiff M, Goldman A, et al. Selective costimulation modulation using abatacept in patients with active rheumatoid arthritis while receiving etanercept: a randomised clinical trial. Ann Rheum Dis 2007;66(2):228–34.

62. Simon TA, Askling J, Lacaille D, et al. Infections requiring hospitalization in the abatacept clinical development program: an epidemiological assessment. Arthritis Res Ther 2010;12(2):R67.

63. Bigbee CL, Gonchoroff DG, Vratsanos G, et al. Abatacept treatment does not exacerbate chronic *Mycobacterium tuberculosis* infection in mice. Arthritis Rheum 2007;56(8):2557–65.

64. Schiff M, Keiserman M, Codding C, et al. Efficacy and safety of abatacept or infliximab vs placebo in ATTEST: a phase III, multi-centre, randomised, double-blind, placebo-controlled study in patients with rheumatoid arthritis and an inadequate response to methotrexate. Ann Rheum Dis 2008;67(8):1096–103.

65. Schiff MH, Kremer JM, Jahreis A, et al. Integrated safety in tocilizumab clinical trials. Arthritis Res Ther 2011;13(5):R141.

66. Koike T, Harigai M, Inokuma S, et al. Postmarketing surveillance of tocilizumab for rheumatoid arthritis in Japan: interim analysis of 3881 patients. Ann Rheum Dis 2011;70(12):2148–51.

67. Fleischmann RM, Tesser J, Schiff MH, et al. Safety of extended treatment with anakinra in patients with rheumatoid arthritis. Ann Rheum Dis 2006;65(8): 1006–12.

68. Genovese MC, Cohen S, Moreland L, et al. Combination therapy with etanercept and anakinra in the treatment of patients with rheumatoid arthritis who have been treated unsuccessfully with methotrexate. Arthritis Rheum 2004;50(5):1412–9.

69. Maeshima K, Yamaoka K, Kubo S, et al. The JAK inhibitor tofacitinib regulates synovitis through inhibition of interferon-gamma and interleukin-17 production by human CD4 + T cells. Arthritis Rheum 2012;64(6):1790–8.

70. Zerbini CA, Lomonte AB. Tofacitinib for the treatment of rheumatoid arthritis. Expert Rev Clin Immunol 2012;8(4):319–31.

71. Tanaka Y, Suzuki M, Nakamura H, et al, Tofacitinib Study Investigators. Phase II study of tofacitinib (CP-690,550) combined with methotrexate in patients with rheumatoid arthritis and an inadequate response to methotrexate. Arthritis Care Res (Hoboken) 2011;63(8):1150–8.

72. Kremer JM, Cohen S, Wilkinson BE, et al. A phase IIb dose-ranging study of the oral JAK inhibitor tofacitinib (CP-690,550) versus placebo in combination with background methotrexate in patients with active rheumatoid arthritis and an inadequate response to methotrexate alone. Arthritis Rheum 2012;64(4):970–81.

73. Doran MF, Crowson CS, Pond GR, et al. Predictors of infection in rheumatoid arthritis. Arthritis Rheum 2002;46(9):2294–300.

74. Dubost JJ, Soubrier M, De Champs C, et al. No changes in the distribution of organisms responsible for septic arthritis over a 20 year period. Ann Rheum Dis 2002;61(3):267–9.

75. Kollef MH, Shorr A, Tabak YP, et al. Epidemiology and outcomes of health-care-associated pneumonia: results from a large US database of culture-positive pneumonia. Chest 2005;128(6):3854–62.

76. Targonski PV, Poland GA. Pneumococcal vaccination in adults: recommendations, trends, and prospects. Cleve Clin J Med 2007;74(6):401–6, 408–10, 413–4.

77. Kapetanovic MC, Saxne T, Sjoholm A, et al. Influence of methotrexate, TNF blockers and prednisolone on antibody responses to pneumococcal polysaccharide vaccine in patients with rheumatoid arthritis. Rheumatology (Oxford) 2006; 45(1):106–11.

78. Available at: http://www.fda.gov/NewsEvents/Newsroom/PressAnnouncements/ucm285431.htm. Accessed August 16, 2012.

79. Available at: http://www.aafp.org/online/en/home/publications/news/news-now/health-of-the-public/20120626juneacipmtg.html. Accessed August 16, 2012.

80. Oren S, Mandelboim M, Braun-Moscovici Y, et al. Vaccination against influenza in patients with rheumatoid arthritis: the effect of rituximab on the humoral response. Ann Rheum Dis 2008;67(7):937–41.

81. Fomin I, Caspi D, Levy V, et al. Vaccination against influenza in rheumatoid arthritis: the effect of disease modifying drugs, including TNF alpha blockers. Ann Rheum Dis 2006;65(2):191–4.

82. Winthrop KL, Calabrese LH. Let the fog be lifted: screening for hepatitis B virus before biological therapy. Ann Rheum Dis 2011;70(10):1701–3.

83. Vassilopoulos D, Calabrese LH. Management of rheumatic disease with comorbid HBV or HCV infection. Nat Rev Rheumatol 2012;8(6):348–57.

84. Oxman MN, Levin MJ, Shingles Prevention Study Group. Vaccination against herpes zoster and postherpetic neuralgia. J Infect Dis 2008;197(Suppl 2): S228–36.

85. Zhang J, Xie F, Delzell E, et al. Association between vaccination for herpes zoster and risk of herpes zoster infection among older patients with selected immune-mediated diseases. JAMA 2012;308(1):43–9.

86. Winthrop KL, Siegel JN, Jereb J, et al. Tuberculosis associated with therapy against tumor necrosis factor alpha. Arthritis Rheum 2005;52(10):2968–74.

87. Beglinger C, Dudler J, Mottet C, et al. Screening for tuberculosis infection before the initiation of an anti-TNF-alpha therapy. Swiss Med Wkly 2007;137(43–44):620–2.

88. Winthrop KL, Weinblatt M, Daley CL. You can't always get what you want, but if you try sometimes (with two tests–TST and IGRA for tuberculosis), you get what you need. Ann Rheum Dis 2012. [Epub ahead of print].
89. Griffith DE, Aksamit T, Brown-Elliott BA, et al. An official ATS/IDSA statement: diagnosis, treatment, and prevention of nontuberculous mycobacterial diseases. Am J Respir Crit Care Med 2007;175(4):367–416.
90. van Ingen J, Boeree M, Janssen M, et al. Pulmonary *Mycobacterium szulgai* infection and treatment in a patient receiving anti-tumor necrosis factor therapy. Nat Clin Pract Rheumatol 2007;3(7):414–9.
91. Komano Y, Tanaka M, Nanki T, et al. Incidence and risk factors for serious infection in patients with rheumatoid arthritis treated with tumor necrosis factor inhibitors: a report from the Registry of Japanese Rheumatoid Arthritis Patients for Longterm Safety. J Rheumatol 2011;38(7):1258–64.
92. Salmon-Ceron D, Tubach F, Lortholary O, et al. Drug-specific risk of non-tuberculosis opportunistic infections in patients receiving anti-TNF therapy reported to the 3-year prospective French RATIO registry. Ann Rheum Dis 2011;70(4):616–23.
93. Greenberg JD, Reed G, Kremer JM, et al. Association of methotrexate and tumour necrosis factor antagonists with risk of infectious outcomes including opportunistic infections in the CORRONA registry. Ann Rheum Dis 2010;69(2):380–6.
94. Winthrop KL, Baxter R, Liu L, et al. The reliability of diagnostic coding and laboratory data to identify tuberculosis and nontuberculous mycobacterial disease among rheumatoid arthritis patients using anti-tumor necrosis factor therapy. Pharmacoepidemiol Drug Saf 2011;20(3):229–35.
95. McDonald JR, Zeringue AL, Caplan L, et al. Herpes zoster risk factors in a national cohort of veterans with rheumatoid arthritis. Clin Infect Dis 2009;48(10):1364–71.

Perioperative Drug Safety in Patients with Rheumatoid Arthritis

Susan M. Goodman, MD[a], Stephen Paget, MD[a,b],*

KEYWORDS

- Perioperative rheumatoid arthritis • Drug safety • Total joint arthroplasty
- Orthopedic surgery

KEY POINTS

- Although the rates of total joint arthroplasty (TJA) have increased markedly in the general population, fewer patients with rheumatoid arthritis (RA) undergo joint surgery.
- Given the fact that most patients with RA are being treated with disease-modifying antirheumatic drugs, those hospitalized for orthopedic surgery, particularly arthroplasty, are on drug regimens that can affect the outcome of surgery and therefore must be factored into the care plan.
- Perioperative management decisions for patients with RA must balance the potential conflict between wound healing and infection risk against ongoing disease control and the ability to participate in postoperative rehabilitation routines that are critical for TJA outcome.
- Patients with RA who undergo orthopedic surgery for joint destruction typically have more severe disease and are those for whom therapy has failed.

INTRODUCTION

Contemporary rheumatoid arthritis (RA) has become milder, and fewer patients develop erosive, destructive disease than described in historical cohorts. This change is theorized to be associated with changes in biology and is clearly associated with a more aggressive treatment paradigm involving the increasingly widespread early use of potent disease-modifying antirheumatic drugs (DMARDs).[1] Population studies show a decrease in all-cause hospitalizations for RA over the past decade, including a decrease in admissions for arthroplasty.[2]

Although the rates of total joint arthroplasty (TJA) have increased markedly in the general population,[3] fewer patients with RA undergo joint surgery. The rate of hip

---

[a] Rheumatology Division, Hospital For Special Surgery, New York, NY, USA; [b] Internal Medicine, Weill Cornell Medical College, New York, NY, USA
* Corresponding author.
E-mail address: pagets@hss.edu

Rheum Dis Clin N Am 38 (2012) 747–759
http://dx.doi.org/10.1016/j.rdc.2012.08.006
0889-857X/12/$ – see front matter © 2012 Elsevier Inc. All rights reserved.

surgery in patients with RA has remained stable, soft tissue procedures have decreased, and, paradoxically, knee surgery has increased, with the latter attributable to osteoarthritis and the increase in obesity in patients with RA. Given the fact that most patients with RA are being treated with DMARDs, those hospitalized for orthopedic surgery, and particularly arthroplasty, are on drug regimens that can affect the outcome of the surgery and therefore must be factored into the care plan. Perioperative management decisions regarding patients with RA must balance the potential conflict between wound healing and infection risk against ongoing disease control and the ability to participate in postoperative rehabilitation routines that are critical for TJA outcome. The significant expense in both health care dollars and individual morbidity of TJA infection further magnifies the importance of this conflict.

Patients with RA who undergo orthopedic surgery for joint destruction typically have more severe disease and are those for whom therapy has failed. From 2005 to 2007, the total knee arthroplasty rate was 220 per 100,000 patient years, a remarkable increase from 31 per 100,000 patient years between 1971 and 1976, with an estimated 3% to 4% performed in patients with RA.[3] Predictors of severe disease logically overlap with predictors of TJA, and have been identified from large cohort studies. These include poor function on the Health Assessment Questionnaire, persistent elevations of erythrocyte sedimentation rate and C-reactive protein (CRP), and the presence of nodules, extra-articular disease, and erosions within the first year of disease.[4,5] Among patients undergoing a first TJA, 25% will undergo a second TJA within the following year, and 50% will undergo a second TJA within 7 years.[6] Mortality reports are inconsistent, however. Although an increase in mortality has been reported in one cohort of patients with RA undergoing arthroplasty,[7] population-based studies have failed to confirm this increase.[8]

Although the more widespread use of DMARDs has contributed to the improved outcome and a less severe course for RA, the risks and benefits of DMARD use in the perioperative period have not been well defined. DMARD use has increased in patients undergoing orthopedic surgery, as it has in the general RA population. Among patients with RA who underwent orthopedic surgery, only 30% with RA onset between 1980 and 1994 received methotrexate, compared with 64% of those with onset of RA between 1995 and 2007. None in the early cohort had received biologic response modifiers, whereas 20% in the later cohort had. Corticosteroid use was also increased in the later cohort, increasing from 51% to 81%.[7] Given the potent immune suppressant characteristics of these medications, understandable concerns have been raised regarding perioperative use. Patients with RA intrinsically have a 2-fold increased risk of infections when not taking an immunosuppressive drug. Moreover, RA confers an infection risk 2 to 4 times that of osteoarthritis in patients undergoing arthroplasty,[9,10] and RA with high disease activity has also been shown to increase the risk of infection.[11] Concerns about the increased risk of surgical site infection and delayed wound healing have led many clinicians to withhold disease-modifying drugs preoperatively. This approach may lead to a postoperative flare, a reality that may make compliance with postoperative rehabilitation regimens more difficult. Additionally, postoperative flare has an unknown impact on long-term orthopedic outcomes. Loss of efficacy of an established medication regimen is an additional concern when medications are withheld before surgery. Recommendations for medication management in patients with RA undergoing surgery are extrapolated from the experiences of orthopedists, rheumatologists, and gastrointestinal surgeons operating on patients with inflammatory bowel disease. The unique concerns associated with infection risk when orthopedic devices are implanted into a susceptible patient, and the distinctive demands of postoperative orthopedic rehabilitation necessitate a unique approach to patients with RA undergoing orthopedic surgery. This article considers the recent literature on the topic of perioperative use of medications commonly used in RA and assesses the strengths and weaknesses of the available data.

CORTICOSTEROIDS

Corticosteroids have a broad and strong impact on innate and adaptive immunity, leading to the general concept that no other immunosuppressive drug is associated with a higher risk for any type of infection. Corticosteroid use remains highly prevalent in patients with RA, and has well-recognized effects on symptom control, with more recent studies showing a disease-modifying effect.[12] A recent study assessing corticosteroid use found that although 35% of 12,749 patients with RA were current corticosteroid users, 65% had used corticosteroids at any point in their lifetime, and use varied with disease severity. Poorer outcomes were more common in current than in prior corticosteroid users, with increases in rates of mortality (5.7% vs 2.6%), work disability (28.4% vs 17.2%), and TJA (18.5% vs 13%).[13] Infection risk varied with cumulative and absolute doses. The risk of infection in a current user of prednisolone, 5 mg, was 30% after 3 months of therapy, 46% after 6 months of therapy, and 100% after 3 years of therapy.[14]

Infection remains strongly associated with corticosteroid use, even at low doses, with a dose-dependant increase in risk.[15] In addition to their use before admission, corticosteroids may be incorporated into multimodal regimens for postoperative pain and nausea control.[16] The widespread preference for corticosteroid use over traditional and biologic DMARDs in the perioperative period to prevent flare warrants reevaluation.

Given the prevalence of corticosteroid use in RA, and the association of corticosteroid use with disease severity, many patients with RA undergoing orthopedic surgery are likely to be current corticosteroid users. Because prolonged use of corticosteroids will predictably suppress the hypothalamic-pituitary-adrenal (HPA) axis, many patients are given supraphysiologic doses ("stress doses") of steroids to support the HPA axis during the stress of surgery and prevent catastrophic hypotension. Careful study has raised questions about this practice, however. When patients who had adrenal insufficiency based on corticotropin testing were given either their daily steroid dose plus saline plus excess corticosteroids or their usual daily dose plus saline alone, no hemodynamic difference was seen between the groups.[17]

In a classic study, 21 of 41 patients with RA undergoing synovectomy were chronically treated with corticosteroids, and 16 of these 21 had adrenal insufficiency on testing. These patients were compared with the 20 patients with RA who had not been treated with corticosteroids who served as controls. Corticosteroid therapy was stopped 18 hours before surgery in 20 patients and 48 hours before surgery in 1 patient. Although the blood pressure in the corticosteroid-treated patients was lower than that in patients who had not received corticosteroids, the differences were not significant, except in the patient whose corticosteroid was discontinued 48 hours before surgery. Hypotension in that patient responded promptly to intravenous administration of corticosteroids.[18]

Additional studies have confirmed the safety of administering patients' usual daily dose of steroid only in the setting of major orthopedic procedures and allograft nephrectomy.[19–21] Reviews of the available literature support the administration of the usual daily dose of steroid during major surgery, and not supraphysiologic doses.[22] Testing the HPA axis does not provide guidance. Results in patients with presumed secondary adrenal insufficiency from prolonged corticosteroid use do not benefit from HPA testing before surgery, because the results do not predict clinical course.

Patients with presumed secondary adrenal insufficiency can be given their usual daily steroid dose on the morning of surgery. Intraoperative hypotension can be easily treated with intravenous hydrocortisone should the need arise. This recommendation does not apply to patients with primary HPA insufficiency, and has not been tested in patients who have received chronic corticosteroids during childhood development, such as those with juvenile inflammatory arthritis. Perioperative surgical site infections and wound healing may benefit from a more restricted approach to perioperative corticosteroid administration.

METHOTREXATE

Methotrexate has been best studied in the perioperative period. In a prospective study, 388 patients undergoing orthopedic surgery were randomly assigned to either continue or discontinue methotrexate, and also compared with patients who were not taking methotrexate at the time of surgery. The incidence of surgical complications or infections was highest (15%) in the group that discontinued methotrexate, compared with 2% in the group continuing methotrexate. Flares were also high in the group discontinuing methotrexate.[23] This finding has been confirmed in multiple other prospective and retrospective studies.[24–26] More recently, 65 cases from the original 388 patients studied were followed up, and none had developed late infection, leading the authors to conclude that late infections are not increased in methotrexate users either.[27] Although the doses used in these studies (10–15 mg/wk) may not be as high as the doses currently being used (20–25 mg/wk), continuing methotrexate during the perioperative period seems safe, without detrimental effects on wound healing or infection rate. Alternative treatment regimens using corticosteroids to replace methotrexate in the perioperative period lack evidence in the literature and may be less safe. Patients with a significant comorbidity burden, such as those with diabetes or renal functional impairment, may warrant a different approach to perioperative methotrexate dosing, although no studies support a more conservative approach.

LEFLUNOMIDE

Leflunomide is a DMARD with proven efficacy comparable to methotrexate in controlling inflammation and preventing ongoing radiographic damage in patients with RA.[28] The prevalence of infection associated with leflunomide use is not as clear, however. Two small studies addressing perioperative risk reached opposite results, one suggesting no increase in infection and wound healing complications, and the other reporting a significant increase in perioperative complications.[29,30] A larger retrospective audit of 171 patients taking leflunomide suggested a small increase in infection, particularly significant in patients who had severe disease and those who were also receiving methotrexate or corticosteroids. Patients in this report also had rapidly progressive infections that responded poorly to appropriate antibiotic therapy.[31] The prolonged elimination half-life of leflunomide also differentiates it from other traditional DMARDs. It therefore seems prudent to withhold leflunomide preoperatively, and consider a prolonged (2-week) period off-drug before surgery in patients with other significant infection-related risk factors, such as diabetes or corticosteroid use.

BIOLOGIC THERAPY
Tumor Necrosis Factor Inhibitors

The addition of tumor necrosis factor inhibitors (TNFis) to the RA armamentarium has completely revolutionized the expectations and goals of RA therapy. Patients frequently experience remission, an outcome that was unanticipated as recently as the past decade. Although these potent immunosuppressant medications share an unequivocal increase in the risk of serious infection, much of the initial published experience was biased, because the more severe RA cases were the early recipients of these novel drugs. These patients frequently concurrently received corticosteroids or other immunosuppressants.[32,33] Later, meticulous analyses began to raise questions about the infection risk associated with TNFi use, and the importance of comorbidities and use of medications such as corticosteroids has again been noted.[34] Although an overall risk of infection is consistently associated with TNFi and corticosteroid use,[35] the specific risk of infection in patients undergoing arthroplasty is less clear, because most studies are either too small to detect infection or are retrospective studies or case series.[36–38] Although TNFi use during wound healing may be of benefit, concerns regarding the potential for heightened infection risk have understandably taken precedence. Current guidelines developed by various national rheumatic disease societies, such as the American College of Rheumatology (ACR) and the British Society for Rheumatology, recommend stopping TNFi use 1 to 4 weeks before surgery, proportional to the drugs' half-lives. Until studies clearly delineate the comorbidities and concurrent medications that contribute to the increase in risk, caution dictates holding these agents preoperatively. Given the disparity in national society guidelines, caution would suggest adherence to the more rigorous guidelines for patients with other infection risk factors, such as diabetes, older age, lung or cardiac disease, or concurrent therapy with corticosteroids. Short-term prophylaxis for bacterial infection after arthroplasty can also include implant fixation with antibiotic-laden cement when appropriate.

Rituximab

Rituximab is a monoclonal antibody that targets the CD20 B-cell antigen and is useful and approved for patients with RA who have not had a satisfactory response to TNFi use, and has shown efficacy in both symptom control and radiographic progression.[39,40] Compared with TNFi, rituximab is associated with a lower risk for bacterial infections, which are the primary concern in perioperative management, although the presence of low immunoglobulin levels in a small proportion of patients raises the infection risk. Rituximab has been shown to be safe in patients with prior recurrent bacterial infections,[41] which is reassuring when considering TJA, given its prolonged duration of action. The association with reactivation of Jakob-Creutzfeldt disease and resultant progressive multifocal leukoencephalopathy, and for hepatitis B reactivation, are notable but have little impact on perioperative management. Preoperative screening of immunoglobulin levels in patients at high risk for surgical site infection might be considered, but no studies support that approach and no therapy exists to modify an identified increased risk. Administration of intravenous immunoglobulin as a preoperative preventive regimen would be experimental, although implant fixation with antibiotic-laden cement, when appropriate, should be considered.

Abatacept

Abatacept, a human fusion protein of CTLA-4 and immunoglobulin, is an effective medication for the treatment of RA that acts through down-regulating T-cell activation.[42,43] The risk of infection in patients treated with abatacept is not significantly increased over baseline nonbiologic-treated RA.[44] Abatacept is administered either as a monthly infusion or a weekly subcutaneous injection, and conservative timing of surgery should be at the end of the dose cycle.

Tocilizumab

Tocilizumab is a humanized monoclonal antibody that targets the IL-6 receptor. It can be used either as monotherapy or in conjunction with other DMARDs, and is effective in treating the signs and symptoms of RA, and in slowing radiographic progression. Infection rates attributed to tocilizumab are comparable to those associated with other biologic DMARDs.[45] A retrospective study that compared 161 orthopedic surgical patients who had received tocilizumab with those taking other DMARDs found no increase in infection, which was seen in 3 patients. Wound healing seemed delayed in 20 cases. Additionally, the usual elevation of CRP and temperature associated with surgery was not seen, a finding confirmed in another retrospective series of orthopedic cases treated with tocilizumab. Flares of RA were also seen, and in these cases the CRP was elevated.[46,47] The direct effect of tocilizumab on temperature and CRP, observed in multiple settings, may lead to a delay in diagnosing infection in the postoperative period. Although clinical complaints may raise the index of suspicion for an infectious complication, these patients may be also receiving analgesics, as would be appropriate in the postoperative setting, further decreasing the clinical clues of a complication. As with other biologic DMARDs, discontinuing tocilizumab before surgery based on the drug half-life of 11 to 13 days is a safe approach to perioperative therapy. Additionally, heightened vigilance for complications is required given the absence of cues, such as fever.

Tofacitinib

This oral DMARD is likely to be approved soon for use in RA, and has shown efficacy in control of symptoms and in slowing radiographic progression (Kremer). The Janus activated kinase 3 (JAK3) has an essential role in cytokine signal transduction, and regulates lymphocyte differentiation and survival.[48] Adverse events reported in early trials include anemia, neutropenia, and upper respiratory infections.[49] Insufficient information is currently available to make recommendations regarding perioperative management.

Nonsteroidal Anti-Inflammatory Drugs

Nonsteroidal anti-inflammatory drugs (NSAIDs) are included in the 2012 recommendations for the management of osteoarthritis of the hip, knee, as well as therapy for RA, and although recognition of potential associated cardiac, renal, and vascular toxicity has prompted caution. NSAIDs are widely used for this indication.[50] Osteoarthritis is the diagnosis in most patients admitted for arthroplasty, and therefore patients presenting for surgery frequently list NSAIDs among their preoperative medications.[51] NSAIDs are widely used postoperatively in multimodal pain management regimens to decrease narcotic use and adverse narcotic effects.[52,53] An additional use is to prevent heterotopic ossification, with new bone formation at the site of surgical trauma that may lead to long-term functional limitation and pain.[54] Significant concerns exist regarding preoperative NSAID use, however, including bleeding risk, cardiovascular risk, and risk of poor bony ingrowth of noncemented prostheses and a decrease in bone fusion rates.

    Excessive bleeding may theoretically result when NSAIDs are continued up to the time of surgery, because of the reversible effect of NSAIDs on platelet function. Evidence supporting a significant increase in blood loss with preoperative administration of nonselective NSAIDs compared with cyclooxygenase-2 (COX-2)–selective NSAIDs include studies showing that indomethacin was associated with 17% more blood loss than meloxicam[55]; diclofenac was associated with 32% greater blood loss than rofecoxib[56]; and ibuprofen was associated with 45% greater blood loss.[57]

Because the effect of NSAIDs on platelet function is reversible, simply discontinuing the medications using a formula based on doubling the drug half-life provides adequate safety. Lower extremity arthroplasty is typically performed under either hypotensive anesthesia or tourniquet, which diminishes blood loss and therefore lessens the potential significance of blood loss associated with NSAID use. In fact, some orthopedists at the authors' institution continue NSAIDs through surgery.

NSAIDs may also contribute to postoperative bleeding from interactions with warfarin anticoagulants. Enzymes in the cytochrome P450 (CYP) pathway play a key role in the metabolism of both warfarin and NSAIDs, and enzyme variants have been linked to excessive anticoagulation. Among 100 patients undergoing total hip arthroplasty, 11 of 30 who were heterozygous for a CYP variant had an international normalized ratio (INR) greater than 4.9. Only those who had received NSAIDs had significant elevations of INR.[58] In the outpatient setting, a cohort study showed a significant increase in risk with an INR greater than 6 when patients anticoagulated with warfarin had CYP variants and received NSAIDs.[59] Additionally, the effect of inhibiting platelet aggregation and decreasing traditional vitamin K–dependant clotting factors with warfarin is additive. Given the role of warfarin as a cornerstone of thromboembolism prophylaxis after TJA, avoiding NSAIDs during the period of prophylaxis and careful monitoring of INR are strongly recommended for all patients on warfarin given the high frequency of the CYP allelic variant and multiple other potential interactions.

Cardiovascular risk associated with NSAIDs has been well described; COX-2 inhibitors were prescribed with the intent of avoiding COX-1–mediated gastrointestinal toxicity while abrogating COX-2–mediated pain and inflammation. Subsequent large studies have shown an increase in cardiovascular events and thrombotic events with NSAIDs, particularly COX-2 inhibitors.[60–62] Recently, this effect was elucidated in a model in which deletion of the COX-2 gene in endothelial cells resulted in decreased production of prostacyclin (PGI_2), which decreases platelet aggregation, vasoconstriction, and thrombosis, through showing a decrease in the excretion of a PGI_2 metabolite. Nitrous oxide, a potent protective vasodilator, was also reduced.[63] Although the theoretical risks are significant, when troponin levels were obtained on 1518 (14%) of 10,873 patients undergoing arthroplasty, elevations were seen in 0.8 of 9831 patients who received NSAIDs, compared with 1.8 of 1042 patients who did not, showing no increase in cardiovascular events after arthroplasty with a mean duration of therapy of 3 days.[64] A cautious approach to NSAIDs and COX-2s would include withholding COX-2s in the perioperative period in patients at high risk for cardiovascular events, and treating for a short duration when NSAIDs or COX-2s are indicated.

Bony ingrowth inhibition by NSAIDs and COX-2s in noncemented prostheses is concerning, given the role of prostaglandins in osteoblast and osteoclast regulation. Although in vitro studies have shown a decrease in bony ingrowth in animal models, short-term administration of COX-2s do not have the deleterious effect on bone that 6-week courses of therapy have.[65,66] In vivo studies assessing prosthesis migration via radiostereometric analysis has not shown a difference in patients randomized to receive either celecoxib versus placebo after TJA.[67] Using a model in which tetracycline labeling allows measurement of bony ingrowth into plugs during staged total knee arthroplasty, no difference in bony ingrowth in patients treated with celecoxib versus placebo could be shown.[68] The clinical concern regarding fixation of noncemented prostheses has not been substantiated, and therefore NSAIDs and COX2s can be used after arthroplasty for short-term pain relief without concern for bony in growth.

Table 1
Common DMARDs used in RA

Medication	Impact on Immune System	Recommended Perioperative Actions	Pharmacologic Half-Life
Corticosteroids	Immunosuppressive via innate and adaptive immune system	Minimize exposure with lowest possible dose necessary to maintain hemodynamic stability	Variable
Methotrexate	Inhibits lymphocyte proliferation, increases adenosine release, anti-inflammatory	Maintain usual dose if under 20 mg/wk; consider lower dose if high-risk	3–15 h
Leflunomide	Inhibits pyrimidine synthesis, immunosuppressive	If high-risk, stop 2 wk before surgery	>14 d
Rituximab	Binds B-cell surface antigen CD20	If high-risk, consider checking immunoglobulin levels	>76 h, effect lasts >6 mo
Abatacept	Modulates T-cell activation; costimulatory blocker	Last dose 4 wk before surgery	13.1–14.3 d
Tocilizumab	Binds IL-6 receptor, reduces inflammation, and alters immune response	Last dose 4 wk before surgery	11–13 d
TNF inhibitors	Bind and inhibit TNF-α, alter immune response, anti-inflammatory	Last dose: double half-life	Infliximab: 8–9.5 d Adalimumab: 14 d Etanercept: 102 h Golimumab: 14 d Certolizumab pegol: 14 d

OSTEOPOROSIS THERAPY

Although estrogen is used less frequently in the treatment and prevention of osteoporosis, it should be discontinued in the RA setting because of its well-recognized increased risk for thromboembolism. Similar concerns exist for tamoxifen and raloxifene.

Bisphosphonates are commonly used to treat osteoporosis, and are frequently encountered preoperatively. Revision surgery may be indicated as a result of periprosthetic bone loss with osteolysis and loosening, but some evidence shows that bisphosphonates may slow this process. Bisphosphonates have been associated with a decrease in all-cause revision, and have increased implant survival.[69,70] No prospective studies have confirmed this finding, however.

SUMMARY

The expansion of therapeutic options for the therapy of RA has improved the functional, quality of life, and radiographic outcomes for patients with RA, although immunomodulatory and immunosuppressive effects may increase the potential for complications related to infection risk or wound healing after orthopedic surgery. Additionally, medications without significant effects on the immune system, such as NSAIDs, may have consequences in terms of bleeding or cardiovascular disease.

Although the benefits of these medications have been remarkable, increased vigilance is required, particularly in the perioperative period (**Table 1**).

REFERENCES

1. Pincus T, Sokka T, Kautiainen H. Patients seen for standard rheumatoid arthritis care have significantly better articular, radiographic, laboratory, and functional status in 2000 than in 1985. Arthritis Rheum 2005;52(4):1009–19.
2. Weiss RJ, Stark A, Wick MC, et al. Orthopaedic surgery of the lower limbs in 49,802 rheumatoid arthritis patients: results from the Swedish National Inpatient Registry during 1987 to 2001. Ann Rheum Dis 2006;65(3):335–41.
3. Singh JA, Vessely MB, Harmsen WS, et al. A population-based study of trends in the use of total hip and total knee arthroplasty, 1969-2008. Mayo Clin Proc 2010; 85(10):898–904.
4. Kapetanovic MC, Lindqvist E, Saxne T, et al. Orthopaedic surgery in patients with rheumatoid arthritis over 20 years: prevalence and predictive factors of large joint replacement. Ann Rheum Dis 2008;67(10):1412–6.
5. Massardo L, Gabriel SE, Crowson CS, et al. A population based assessment of the use of orthopedic surgery in patients with rheumatoid arthritis. J Rheumatol 2002;29(1):52–6.
6. Wolfe F, Zwillich SH. The long-term outcomes of rheumatoid arthritis: a 23-year prospective, longitudinal study of total joint replacement and its predictors in 1,600 patients with rheumatoid arthritis. Arthritis Rheum 1998;41(6):1072–82.
7. Shourt CA, Crowson CS, Gabriel SE, et al. Orthopedic surgery among patients with rheumatoid arthritis 1980-2007: a population-based study focused on surgery rates, sex, and mortality. J Rheumatol 2012;39(3):481–5.
8. Singh JA, Kundukulam J, Riddle DL, et al. Early postoperative mortality following joint arthroplasty: a systematic review. J Rheumatol 2011;38(7):1507–13.
9. Bongartz T, Halligan CS, Osmon DR, et al. Incidence and risk factors of prosthetic joint infection after total hip or knee replacement in patients with rheumatoid arthritis. Arthritis Rheum 2008;59(12):1713–20.
10. Giles JT, Bartlett SJ, Gelber AC, et al. Tumor necrosis factor inhibitor therapy and risk of serious postoperative orthopedic infection in rheumatoid arthritis. Arthritis Rheum 2006;55(2):333–7.
11. Au K, Reed G, Curtis JR, et al. High disease activity is associated with an increased risk of infection in patients with rheumatoid arthritis. Ann Rheum Dis 2011;70(5):785–91.
12. Bakker MF, Jacobs JW, Welsing PM, et al. Low-dose prednisone inclusion in a methotrexate-based, tight control strategy for early rheumatoid arthritis: a randomized trial. Ann Intern Med 2012;156(5):329–39.
13. Caplan L, Wolfe F, Russell AS, et al. Corticosteroid use in rheumatoid arthritis: prevalence, predictors, correlates, and outcomes. J Rheumatol 2007;34(4):696–705.
14. Dixon WG, Abrahamowicz M, Beauchamp ME, et al. Immediate and delayed impact of oral glucocorticoid therapy on risk of serious infection in older patients with rheumatoid arthritis: a nested case-control analysis. Ann Rheum Dis 2012; 71(7):1128–33.
15. Grijalva CG, Chen L, Delzell E, et al. Initiation of tumor necrosis factor-alpha antagonists and the risk of hospitalization for infection in patients with autoimmune diseases. JAMA 2011;306(21):2331–9.
16. Ayalon O, Liu S, Flics S, et al. A multimodal clinical pathway can reduce length of stay after total knee arthroplasty. HSS J 2011;7(1):9–15.

17. Glowniak JV, Loriaux DL. A double-blind study of perioperative steroid require-
    ments in secondary adrenal insufficiency. Surgery 1997;121(2):123–9.
18. Jasani MK, Freeman PA, Boyle JA, et al. Cardiovascular and plasma cortisol
    responses to surgery in corticosteroid-treated R. A. patients. Acta Rheumatol
    Scand 1968;14(1):65–70.
19. Bromberg JS, Alfrey EJ, Barker CF, et al. Adrenal suppression and steroid supple-
    mentation in renal transplant recipients. Transplantation 1991;51(2):385–90.
20. Friedman RJ, Schiff CF, Bromberg JS. Use of supplemental steroids in patients
    having orthopaedic operations. J Bone Joint Surg Am 1995;77(12):1801–6.
21. Shapiro R, Carroll PB, Tzakis AG, et al. Adrenal reserve in renal transplant recip-
    ients with cyclosporine, azathioprine, and prednisone immunosuppression.
    Transplantation 1990;49(5):1011–3.
22. Marik PE, Varon J. Requirement of perioperative stress doses of corticosteroids:
    a systematic review of the literature. Arch Surg 2008;143(12):1222–6.
23. Grennan DM, Gray J, Loudon J, et al. Methotrexate and early postoperative
    complications in patients with rheumatoid arthritis undergoing elective ortho-
    paedic surgery. Ann Rheum Dis 2001;60(3):214–7.
24. Murata K, Yasuda T, Ito H, et al. Lack of increase in postoperative complications
    with low-dose methotrexate therapy in patients with rheumatoid arthritis under-
    going elective orthopedic surgery. Mod Rheumatol 2006;16(1):14–9.
25. Loza E, Martinez-Lopez JA, Carmona L. A systematic review on the optimum
    management of the use of methotrexate in rheumatoid arthritis patients in the
    perioperative period to minimize perioperative morbidity and maintain disease
    control. Clin Exp Rheumatol 2009;27(5):856–62.
26. Jain A, Witbreuk M, Ball C, et al. Influence of steroids and methotrexate on wound
    complications after elective rheumatoid hand and wrist surgery. J Hand Surg Am
    2002;27(3):449–55.
27. Sreekumar R, Gray J, Kay P, et al. Methotrexate and post operative complications
    in patients with rheumatoid arthritis undergoing elective orthopaedic surgery–
    a ten year follow-up. Acta Orthop Belg 2011;77(6):823–6.
28. Alcorn N, Saunders S, Madhok R. Benefit-risk assessment of leflunomide: an
    appraisal of leflunomide in rheumatoid arthritis 10 years after licensing. Drug
    Saf 2009;32(12):1123–34.
29. Fuerst M, Mohl H, Baumgartel K, et al. Leflunomide increases the risk of early
    healing complications in patients with rheumatoid arthritis undergoing elective
    orthopedic surgery. Rheumatol Int 2006;26(12):1138–42.
30. Tanaka N, Sakahashi H, Sato E, et al. Examination of the risk of continuous leflu-
    nomide treatment on the incidence of infectious complications after joint arthro-
    plasty in patients with rheumatoid arthritis. J Clin Rheumatol 2003;9(2):115–8.
31. Jenks KA, Stamp LK, O'Donnell JL, et al. Leflunomide-associated infections in
    rheumatoid arthritis. J Rheumatol 2007;34(11):2201–3.
32. Doran MF, Crowson CS, Pond GR, et al. Predictors of infection in rheumatoid
    arthritis. Arthritis Rheum 2002;46(9):2294–300.
33. Curtis JR, Patkar N, Xie A, et al. Risk of serious bacterial infections among rheu-
    matoid arthritis patients exposed to tumor necrosis factor alpha antagonists.
    Arthritis Rheum 2007;56(4):1125–33.
34. Curtis JR, Xi J, Patkar N, et al. Drug-specific and time-dependent risks of bacte-
    rial infection among patients with rheumatoid arthritis who were exposed to tumor
    necrosis factor alpha antagonists. Arthritis Rheum 2007;56(12):4226–7.
35. Greenberg JD, Reed G, Kremer JM, et al. Association of methotrexate and
    tumour necrosis factor antagonists with risk of infectious outcomes including

opportunistic infections in the CORRONA registry. Ann Rheum Dis 2010;69(2): 380–6.

36. Bibbo C, Goldberg JW. Infectious and healing complications after elective ortho-paedic foot and ankle surgery during tumor necrosis factor-alpha inhibition therapy. Foot Ankle Int 2004;25(5):331–5.

37. den Broeder AA, Creemers MC, Fransen J, et al. Risk factors for surgical site infections and other complications in elective surgery in patients with rheumatoid arthritis with special attention for anti-tumor necrosis factor: a large retrospective study. J Rheumatol 2007;34(4):689–95.

38. Ruyssen-Witrand A, Gossec L, Salliot C, et al. Complication rates of 127 surgical procedures performed in rheumatic patients receiving tumor necrosis factor alpha blockers. Clin Exp Rheumatol 2007;25(3):430–6.

39. Haraoui B, Bokarewa M, Kallmeyer I, et al. Safety and effectiveness of rituximab in patients with rheumatoid arthritis following an inadequate response to 1 prior tumor necrosis factor inhibitor: the RESET Trial. J Rheumatol 2011;38(12):2548–56.

40. Tak PP, Rigby W, Rubbert-Roth A, et al. Sustained inhibition of progressive joint damage with rituximab plus methotrexate in early active rheumatoid arthritis: 2-year results from the randomised controlled trial IMAGE. Ann Rheum Dis 2012; 71(3):351–7.

41. Toussirot E, Pertuiset E, Sordet C, et al. Safety of rituximab in rheumatoid arthritis patients with a history of severe or recurrent bacterial infection: observational study of 30 cases in everyday practice. Joint Bone Spine 2010;77(2):142–5.

42. Kremer JM, Genant HK, Moreland LW, et al. Effects of abatacept in patients with methotrexate-resistant active rheumatoid arthritis: a randomized trial. Ann Intern Med 2006;144(12):865–76.

43. Kremer JM, Russell AS, Emery P, et al. Long-term safety, efficacy and inhibition of radiographic progression with abatacept treatment in patients with rheumatoid arthritis and an inadequate response to methotrexate: 3-year results from the AIM trial. Ann Rheum Dis 2011;70(10):1826–30.

44. Simon TA, Askling J, Lacaille D, et al. Infections requiring hospitalization in the abatacept clinical development program: an epidemiological assessment. Arthritis Res Ther 2010;12(2):R67.

45. Bykerk VP, Ostor AJ, Alvaro-Gracia J, et al. Tocilizumab in patients with active rheumatoid arthritis and inadequate responses to DMARDs and/or TNF inhibitors: a large, open-label study close to clinical practice. Ann Rheum Dis, in press.

46. Hirao M, Hashimoto J, Tsuboi H, et al. Laboratory and febrile features after joint surgery in patients with rheumatoid arthritis treated with tocilizumab. Ann Rheum Dis 2009;68(5):654–7.

47. Momohara S, Hashimoto J, Tsuboi H, et al. Analysis of perioperative clinical features and complications after orthopaedic surgery in rheumatoid arthritis patients treated with tocilizumab in a real-world setting: results from the multi-centre TOcilizumab in Perioperative Period (TOPP) study. Mod Rheumatol 2012;34(6):467.

48. Fleischmann R. Novel small-molecular therapeutics for rheumatoid arthritis. Curr Opin Rheumatol 2012;24(3):335–41.

49. Kremer JM, Bloom BJ, Breedveld FC, et al. The safety and efficacy of a JAK inhibitor in patients with active rheumatoid arthritis: results of a double-blind, placebo-controlled phase IIa trial of three dosage levels of CP-690,550 versus placebo. Arthritis Rheum 2009;60(7):1895–905.

50. Hochberg MC, Altman RD, April KT, et al. American College of Rheumatology 2012 recommendations for the use of nonpharmacologic and pharmacologic

therapies in osteoarthritis of the hand, hip, and knee. Arthritis Care Res (Hoboken) 2012;64(4):455–74.

51. Berger A, Bozic K, Stacey B, et al. Patterns of pharmacotherapy and health care utilization and costs prior to total hip or total knee replacement in patients with osteoarthritis. Arthritis Rheum 2011;63(8):2268–75.

52. Meunier A, Lisander B, Good L. Effects of celecoxib on blood loss, pain, and recovery of function after total knee replacement: a randomized placebo-controlled trial. Acta Orthop 2007;78(5):661–7.

53. Reuben SS, Buvenandran A, Katz B, et al. A prospective randomized trial on the role of perioperative celecoxib administration for total knee arthroplasty: improving clinical outcomes. Anesth Analg 2008;106(4):1258–64.

54. Vasileiadis GI, Sioutis IC, Mavrogenis AF, et al. COX-2 inhibitors for the prevention of heterotopic ossification after THA. Orthopedics 2011;34(6):467.

55. Weber EW, Slappendel R, Durieux ME, et al. COX 2 selectivity of non-steroidal anti-inflammatory drugs and perioperative blood loss in hip surgery. A randomized comparison of indomethacin and meloxicam. Eur J Anaesthesiol 2003;20(12):963–6.

56. Li W, Lian YY, Yue WJ, et al. Experimental study of COX-2 selective and traditional non-steroidal anti-inflammatory drugs in total hip replacement. J Int Med Res 2009;37(2):472–8.

57. Slappendel R, Weber EW, Benraad B. Does ibuprofen increase perioperative blood loss during hip arthroplasty? Eur J Anaesthesiol 2002;19(11):829–31.

58. Beinema MJ, de Jong PH, Salden HJ, et al. The influence of NSAIDs on coumarin sensitivity in patients with CYP2C9 polymorphism after total hip replacement surgery. Mol Diagn Ther 2007;11(2):123–8.

59. Visser LE, van Schaik RH, van Vliet M, et al. Allelic variants of cytochrome P450 2C9 modify the interaction between nonsteroidal anti-inflammatory drugs and coumarin anticoagulants. Clin Pharmacol Ther 2005;77(6):479–85.

60. Bombardier C, Laine L, Reicin A, et al. Comparison of upper gastrointestinal toxicity of rofecoxib and naproxen in patients with rheumatoid arthritis. VIGOR Study Group. N Engl J Med 2000;343(21):1520–8.

61. Bresalier RS, Sandler RS, Quan H, et al. Cardiovascular events associated with rofecoxib in a colorectal adenoma chemoprevention trial. N Engl J Med 2005; 352(11):1092–102.

62. McGettigan P, Henry D. Cardiovascular risk with non-steroidal anti-inflammatory drugs: systematic review of population-based controlled observational studies. PLoS Med 2011;8(9):e1001098.

63. Yu Y, Ricciotti E, Scalia R, et al. Vascular COX-2 modulates blood pressure and thrombosis in mice. Sci Transl Med 2012;4(132):132ra54.

64. Liu SS, Bae JJ, Bieltz M, et al. Association of perioperative use of nonsteroidal anti-inflammatory drugs with postoperative myocardial infarction after total joint replacement. Reg Anesth Pain Med 2012;37(1):45–50.

65. Goodman S, Ma T, Trindade M, et al. COX-2 selective NSAID decreases bone ingrowth in vivo. J Orthop Res 2002;20(6):1164–9.

66. Goodman SB, Ma T, Mitsunaga L, et al. Temporal effects of a COX-2-selective NSAID on bone ingrowth. J Biomed Mater Res A 2005;72(3):279–87.

67. Meunier A, Aspenberg P, Good L. Celecoxib does not appear to affect prosthesis fixation in total knee replacement: A randomized study using radiostereometry in 50 patients. Acta Orthop 2009;80(1):46–50.

68. Hofmann AA, Bloebaum RD, Koller KE, et al. Does celecoxib have an adverse effect on bone remodeling and ingrowth in humans? Clin Orthop Relat Res 2006;452:200–4.

69. Thillemann TM, Pedersen AB, Mehnert F, et al. Postoperative use of bisphosph-onates and risk of revision after primary total hip arthroplasty: a nationwide pop-ulation-based study. Bone 2010;46(4):946–51.

70. Prieto-Alhambra D, Javaid MK, Judge A, et al. Association between bisphosph-onate use and implant survival after primary total arthroplasty of the knee or hip: population based retrospective cohort study. BMJ 2011;343:d7222.

Malignancy Risks With Biologic Therapies

John J. Cush, MD*, Kathryn H. Dao, MD

KEYWORDS

- Rheumatoid arthritis • Cancer • Biologic agent • Tumor necrosis factor

KEY POINTS

- The management of rheumatoid arthritis (RA) dramatically changed in 1998 with the introduction of etanercept and infliximab for the treatment of RA and Crohn colitis.
- Nine biologic agents are currently in use for treating RA.
- As these agents aim to specifically mitigate the excessive cytokine or cellular activity seen in RA, speculation has grown that the long-term use of these biopharmaceuticals may alter normal immunosurveillance, thereby contributing to an individual's cancer risk.

INTRODUCTION

The management of rheumatoid arthritis (RA) dramatically changed in 1998 with the introduction of etanercept and infliximab, biospecific inhibitors of tumor necrosis factor (TNF) α, for the treatment of RA and Crohn colitis. Since then, 9 biologic agents have met regulatory approval for use in RA. As these agents aim to specifically mitigate the excessive cytokine or cellular activity seen in RA, speculation has grown that the long-term use of these biopharmaceuticals may alter normal immunosurveillance, thereby contributing to an individual's cancer risk. Many studies and reports have speculated on the associations between cancer, RA, and biologic therapy. Whether malignancy is a consequence of rheumatoid inflammation or the therapies used to treat RA has been unclear until recently. This article addresses the growing data on the short- and long-term cancer risks associated with biologic use in RA.

POPULATION CANCER RISK

According to a 2009 cancer statistics review performed by the Surveillance, Epidemiology and End Results (SEER) registry, the U.S. population risk of developing cancer is 41%, with a 21% chance of dying from cancer.[1] The SEER database collects data on

Baylor Research Institute, 9900 N Central Expressway, Suite #550, Dallas, TX 75229, USA
* Corresponding author.
E-mail address: jjcush@gmail.com

Rheum Dis Clin N Am 38 (2012) 761–770
http://dx.doi.org/10.1016/j.rdc.2012.09.006
0889-857X/12/$ – see front matter © 2012 Published by Elsevier Inc.

rheumatic.theclinics.com

cancer events from 17 regional population registries in the United States and represents 28% of the population. The most common cancers involve the skin (affecting 20% of the population), prostate (15% of men), breast (11% of women), lung (6%), and colon (5.3%).[2] Risk factors underlying neoplasia may be constitutive, genetically determined, or enhanced by exogenous factors known to augment risks, such as age, carcinogens, radiation, infection, immunosuppression, or inflammation.

CANCER RISK IN RA

In the prebiologic era, numerous studies showed the overall cancer risk to be the same in RA as in the general population (hence the standardized incidence ratio [SIR] is roughly 1.0). The SIR is calculated by comparing observed with expected cancer rates (usually derived from age- and era-matched populations drawn from the SEER database). Hence, numerous analyses have concluded that there is no overall increase in malignancy in RA.[2–10] However, this summary belies the fact that there is a decreased risk of several malignancies in RA, notably adenocarcinoma of colon and breast cancer (owing to chronic nonsteroidal anti-inflammatory drug use and cyclooxygenase-2 inhibition) (**Table 1**).[4] At the same time, there is a higher risk of certain cancers, including lymphoma, lung cancer (SIR, 1.2–4.0), nonmelanomatous skin cancers (NMSC) (SIR, 1–3), and possibly melanoma and leukemia. Current evidence suggests these are augmented by chronic uncontrolled inflammation and possibly tobacco use.

LYMPHOMA RISK WITH RA AND BIOLOGIC THERAPY
Lymphoma in RA

The age-adjusted incidence rate of lymphoma is 22.5 per 100,000 population per year. The incidence of non-Hodgkin lymphoma has increased in the past 4 decades at a rate of 2% to 3% per year. Increased rates of lymphoma (especially non-Hodgkin lymphoma) in RA seems to be related to advancing age, inflammation manifest as high disease activity (long-standing active RA), and possibly the use of immunosuppressive therapies (azathioprine, alkylating agents) or biologic (anti-TNF) therapies. The lymphoma risk in RA is elevated, with a SIR of between 2 and 11 (2- to 11-fold higher than the general population).[7] Hellgren[5] showed that before the onset of RA, no risk of lymphoma or cancer was evident. However, after disease onset, overall cancer risk remained unchanged while the risk of lymphoma rose, especially after 6 years of active RA. Their study noted an increased 10-year lymphoma risk (relative risk [RR], 1.75; 95% CI, 1.04–2.96). Baecklund and others[6] have shown the

Table 1 Meta-analysis of cancer risk in RA, 2008		
Type of Cancer	SIR	95% CI
Lymphoma	2.08	1.80–2.39
Hodgkin's lymphoma	3.29	2.56–4.22
Non-Hodgkin lymphoma	1.95	1.70–2.24
Lung cancer	1.63	1.43–1.87
Colorectal cancer	0.77	0.65–0.90
Breast cancer	0.84	0.79–0.90
Overall cancer risk	1.05	1.01–1.09

Data from Smitten AL, Simon TA, Hochberg MC, et al. A meta-analysis of the incidence of malignancy in adult patients with rheumatoid arthritis. Arthritis Res Ther 2008;10:R45.

risk of lymphoma to be proportional to the degree and duration of inflammation, with patients with the most severe RA having rates as high as 20- to 71-fold higher than the general population.[9]

Lymphoma With Biologic Therapy

The issue of lymphoma risk with TNF inhibitors arose in 2003 when an analysis by the U.S. Food and Drug Administration (FDA) of the first 6303 patients with RA treated with etanercept, infliximab, and adalimumab found 6 lymphomas in those on TNF inhibitors but none in the placebo-treated controls in the first 6 months of exposure.[7] When patients on placebo went on to receive the TNF inhibitor, 23 total lymphomas were found. Hence, the lymphoma risk was increased for etanercept (SIR, 3.47), infliximab (SIR, 6.4), and adalimumab (SIR, 4.35) (**Table 2**). These elevated SIR values and wide CIs clearly overlap the elevated lymphoma SIR observed in patients with RA from the prebiologic era (**Fig. 1**). These data suggested that patients with RA that was active and severe enough to receive biologic agent assumed an inflammation-dependant risk that was not substantially augmented by use of a TNF inhibitor. Numerous observational studies and metanalyses[7–9] have shown that lymphoma rates in patients with RA are higher than in the general population, and those on biologic agents have the same risk as that seen in patients receiving methotrexate or disease-modifying antirheumatic drugs (DMARDs). A Cochrane meta-analysis examined lymphoma risk in 57 randomized clinical trials involving 22,657 patients treated for a total of 526.3 months with biologics (etanercept, adalimumab, infliximab, golimumab, certolizumab, anakinra, tocilizumab, abatacept, rituximab) and found that patients treated with biologics (0.093%) and controls or those treated with DMARDs (0.091%) had similar lymphoma rates.[10] Their effect estimate for lymphoma was 0.53 (95% CI, 0.17, 1.66) suggesting a risk that was not higher than that seen among patients with RA receiving DMARD therapy alone. The SIR rates from randomized controlled trials of other new biologics have followed those seen with the TNF inhibitors (see **Table 2**). The package inserts for many of these biologics note that more malignancies (especially lymphomas) are noted in patients treated with TNF blockers that in those treated with placebo. The same product labeling estimates the SIR to be between 2 and 6 and

Table 2
SIRs for lymphoma and malignancies in RA on biologics versus the population rate

| Biologic | Registration Randomized Controlled Trials or Package Insert[a] | | |
	Lymphoma SIR (95% CI)	Malignancy SIR (95% CI)	Malignancy Rate Biologic vs Placebo
Abatacept	3.5	0.9 (0.6–1.3)	1.3% vs 1.1%
Adalimumab	4.35 (2.6–10)	1.0 (0.7–1.3)	0.6 vs 0.5 per 100 PY
Anakinra	ND	ND	0.83
Certolizumab	2.06 (0.42–6.02)	0.86 (0.59–1.22)	0.5 vs 0.6 per 100 PY
Etanercept	3.47 (1.6–6.59)	0.98	ND
Golimumab	3.8	Equal to placebo	
Infliximab	6.4 (1.7–16.3)	0.91 (0.53–1.46)	1.31 vs 0.46 per 100 PY
Rituximab	ND	ND	Not increased
Tocilizumab	ND	0.80 (0.77–0.83)	1.32 vs 1.37 per 100 PY

Abbreviations: ND, no data; PY, patient years.
[a] Package insert reporting rates retrieved from ref,[7] manufacturers Web site, or www.dailymed.com (excludes NMSC).

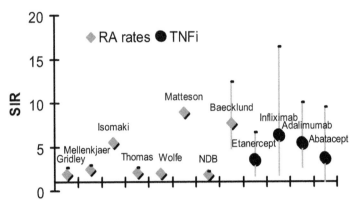

Fig. 1. Lymphoma standardized incidence ratios for RA and RA in Biologics. (*Data from* Cush JJ, Kavanaugh A. ACR Hotline: FDA Meeting March 2003: Update on the safety of new drugs for rheumatoid arthritis. American College of Rheumatology Web site. Available at: http://www.rheumatology.org/publications/hotline/0303TNFL.asp. Accessed November 1, 2012.)

that patients with chronic inflammatory disorders such as RA may be at higher risk for lymphoma (and leukemia) compared with the general population, even in the absence of a biologic. The package inserts state, "the potential role of TNF blocker therapy in the development of malignancies is not known."[2] Many of the RA registries listed in **Fig. 2** have also shown lymphoma rates similar to those reported on the product label. Lastly, no evidence has been seen of increasing risk of cancer or lymphoma over time while on a TNF inhibitor.

Hepatosplenic T-Cell Lymphoma

Hepatosplenic T-cell lymphomas (HSTCLs) have rarely been reported in patients receiving TNF inhibitors. More than 200 HSTCL cases have been documented in the literature. This rare, aggressive, and often fatal malignancy is more frequently found in patients with inflammatory bowel disease (25%) and those who are immunosuppressed or on immunosuppressive drugs.[11] Symptoms include fever, purpura, hepatosplenomegaly, increased hepatic enzymes, and cytopenia, but a notable absence of lymphadenopathy. Although children and young adults (age <30 years) receiving azathioprine or 6-mercaptopurine (for Crohn colitis) are most affected, HSTCL has been rarely reported in those on TNF inhibitors. Six cases (5 deaths) were reported on infliximab, all young with Crohn colitis also receiving thiopurine therapies. Eight cases (4 deaths) were reported on adalimumab, 2 of which were older than 60 years receiving adalimumab for RA.

SOLID TUMOR RISKS FROM RA AND BIOLOGICS

The pattern of malignancies noted in patients with RA treated in the prebiologic era mirrors that seen in the population at large, and includes lung, colorectal, skin, breast, prostate, bladder, ovarian, cervical, and pancreatic cancers. Registration randomized controlled trial data show no increase in overall malignancy risk in patients receiving biologics (see **Table 2**). Moreover, more than 40,000 patients participating in numerous large databases and worldwide RA registries (CORRONA, National Databank, ARTIS, BSRBR, BIOBADASER) have compared the cancer rates between patients treated with TNF inhibitors and DMARDs only and shown consistent rates ($\approx$1%) across

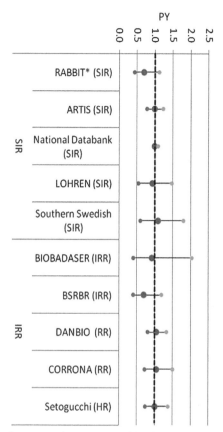

Fig. 2. TNF-inhibitor malignancy risk among worldwide registries and databases. *Includes <5% anakinra patients. IRR, incidence rate ratio; PY, patient-years. (*Adapted from* Cush JJ, Dao KH, Kay J. Does rheumatoid arthritis or biologic therapy increase cancer risk? Drug Safety Quarterly 2012;4(2):1–2. Available at: http://www.rheumatology.org/publications/dsq/dsq_2012_08.pdf#toolbar=1. Accessed September 28, 2012.)

numerous datasets and no increased cancer risk when patients treated with biologics are compared with the general population (reported as SIR rates) or those who are biologic-naïve (reported as hazard ratio, RR, and odds ratio [OR]) (see **Fig. 2**).

Solid tumors (eg, lung, colon, breast, prostate, skin cancer) are the most common cancers occurring in RA and the general population. Cancers known to be increased in RA in the prebiologic era have shown the same pattern with the introduction of biologics. Askling and colleagues[12] examined the rates of solid tumors in RA and found a marginal increase in solid tumors (SIR, 1.05; 95% CI, 1.01–1.08) and higher rates of lung and NMSC. TNF inhibitor use did not augment this risk. Wolfe and Michaud[13] also assessed cancer risk in 13,001 patients in the National Databank for Rheumatic diseases and showed the aforementioned pattern of cancer risk. Biologic use was not associated with an increase risk of solid tumors or lymphoproliferative cancers, but did show an increased risk of NMSC (OR, 1.5; 95% CI, 1.2–1.8) and melanoma (OR, 2.3; 95% CI, 0.9–5.4). Although randomized controlled trials showed abatacept to have similar malignancy rates with placebo (1.3% and 1.1%, respectively), more cases of lung cancer were observed in patients treated with abatacept (n = 4) than in those treated with placebo (n = 0). However, the lung cancer rates in the open-label extension were not different from those in the general population (1.51; 95% CI, 0.80–2.59).[14]

Three unique exploratory clinical trials have been conducted in which unexpected cancers have occurred. More cancer events were observed among patients receiving TNF inhibitors in studies of (1) infliximab in chronic obstructive pulmonary disease,[15] (2) etanercept in Wegener granulomatosis,[16] and (3) golimumab in severe asthma.[17] More solid tumors were observed among patients treated with TNF inhibitors than in those on placebo. Finding these events in small randomized controlled trials was unexpected and carries an uncertain significance.

Melanoma

Melanoma and NMSC have been reported to occur more commonly in patients with RA and those receiving TNF blockers.[9,13] Hence, the standard packaging insert for TNF inhibitors now states that periodic skin examinations should be considered for patients at increased risk for skin cancer. Although the British Society for Rheumatology Biologics Register (BSRBR) 17% melanoma recurrence requires further study and confirmation, not all studies have shown melanoma to be increased in RA. Burmester and colleagues[18] recently reported an elevated melanoma rate in patients with psoriasis (4.37; 95% CI, 1.89–8.61) but not those with RA (SIR, 1.5; 95% CI, 0.84–2.47) receiving adalimumab.

Cancer Risk in Children

Lymphoma and other malignancies have been reported in children and adolescents and adults. The FDA has added language to the product labels for all TNF inhibitors stating that "children receiving TNF-inhibitors are at increased risk of developing cancer, including primarily lymphomas but also rare malignancies associated with immunosuppression and malignancies not usually observed in children and adolescents."[19] This conclusion is based on an FDA analysis (from 2001–2008) that identified 48 cases of malignancies in children receiving TNF inhibitors; half for inflammatory bowel disease (n = 25) and one-third for juvenile arthritis.[20] Nearly 88% were receiving other immunosuppressive therapies, such as azathioprine and methotrexate. The cancers seen in children were different from those seen in adults, with 6 Hodgkin's lymphoma, 7 non-Hodgkin lymphoma, and 10 HSTCL cases. Other malignancies included leukemia,[6] malignant melanoma,[3] leiomyosarcoma, hepatic malignancies, neuroblastoma, and renal cell carcinoma. The denominators for overall drug exposure were provided by the manufacturers, and the expected cancer rates were provided by the SEER pediatric database. Excluding HSTCLs, the observed malignancy rate was 22 per 100,000 patient-years with infliximab and 11 per 100,000 patient-years with etanercept; the expected rate for this population would have been 2.4 per 100,000 patient-years.[20] These data are best understood if it is known what the risk of cancer is in children with juvenile idiopathic arthritis (JIA). Hence, whether a higher cancer rate occurred because of the therapy or the chronic inflammatory condition is unclear. A recent meta-analysis of DMARD use in JIA[21] concluded that information was insufficient to ascribe a cancer risk to therapy. Among 914 patients in randomized controlled trials, no cancers or deaths were seen in those receiving DMARD (including biologic) therapy during the randomized controlled phase of the studies. Of the 4344 patients studied, 7 TNF inhibitor–related cancers (4 lymphoma, 2 thyroid carcinomas, 1 yolk sac carcinoma) and 4 nonbiologic DMARD cancers (all lymphoma) were found.

Bernatsky and colleagues[22] reported no increased risk of cancer in their analysis of 1834 patients from 3 pediatric rheumatology centers in Canada. However, 2 large population-based studies yielded contrasting findings about cancer rates in juvenile arthritis. Nordstrom and colleagues[23] used the PharMetrics Patient-Centric Database to analyze 3605 patients with JIA between 1998 and 2007. They found a cancer incidence rate of 67.0 (95% CI, 1.3–132.5) per 100,000 patient-years for patients with JIA and 23.2 (95% CI, 12.2–34.2) per 100,000 patient-years for those without. Hence, an elevated cancer risk was associated with JIA, with an SIR of 4.0 (95% CI, 2.6–6.0). These findings are similar to 2 other large series reported by Simard and colleagues[24] and Beukelman and colleagues,[25] both showing an elevated cancer risk in 9207 patients with JIA from a Swedish national register (RR, 2.3; 95% CI, 1.2–4.4) and 7812 patients with JIA from the U.S. Medicaid program.

Despite the warnings listing in the TNF inhibitor package inserts, whether children and adolescents exposed to TNF inhibitors have a true risk of developing cancer is unclear. Population-based studies indicate that higher rates of cancer may be expected in JIA. Several unanswered questions remain, including (1) whether the numerators (cancer events) and denominators (patients exposed) provided by the FDA MedWatch system and the manufacturers are accurate, and (2) whether comparisons with the pediatric SEER database may not be temporally correlated, because cancer rates increase each year in children.

CANCER RECURRENCE IN PATIENTS WITH A PRIOR HISTORY OF CANCER

Watson and colleagues[26] analyzed recurrent cancers among 9998 patients with RA treated with anti-TNF therapy at first exposure and 1877 who were biologic-naïve. Patients with RA treated with TNF inhibitor therapy showed the same cancer recurrence rate (20.5 per 1000 patient-years; 95% CI, 7.6–44.5) as those treated with DMARDs (18.2 per 1000 patient-years; 95% CI, 0.5–97.2). In a follow-up study of 13,970 BSRBR patients, Dixon and colleagues[27] found 293 patients with a prior malignancy, and cancer recurrence rates of 25.3 events per 1000 patient-years for those treated with TNF inhibitors and 38.3 events per 1000 patient-years for those on DMARDs, with an adjusted incidence rate ratio of 0.58 (95% CI, 0.23–1.43). Although no overall increase in cancer recurrence was seen, the melanoma recurrence rate (17%) seen among patients treated with TNF inhibitors versus the lack of recurrences among those on DMARDs was concerning. The German Biologics registry (RABBIT) analyzed 122 patients with a history of prior cancer (55 treated with DMARDs and 67 with biologics).[28] The crude incidence rates were similar among those receiving TNF inhibitors (45.5/1000 patient-years; 95% CI, 20.8–86.3), anakinra (32.3/1000 patient-years; 95% CI, 0.8–179.7), and DMARDs (31.4/1000 patient-years; 95% CI, 10.2–73.4). Hence, no significant increase in cancer recurrence rates were seen among these patients (incidence rate ratio, 1.4; 95% CI, 0.5–5.5; $P = .63$).

DEATH FROM CANCER

Despite the data showing that patients with RA have higher mortality rates once they are diagnosed with cancer,[29,30] no evidence shows that biologic use has increased or worsened these mortality rates. Several studies have compared outcomes of patients with RA with neoplasia who continue to receive biologic or DMARD (without biologic) therapy. Patients in the ARTIS/Swedish database who developed cancer were shown to have the same survival rates whether they were exposed to biologics (n = 302) or not (n = 586) (HR, 1.0; 95% CI, 0.8–1.3), even after adjustments for staging, cancer type, or comorbidities.[31] Similarly, Carmona and colleagues[32] and the BIOBADASER Spanish database found that death from cancer was lower among patients treated with TNF inhibitors compared with those treated with DMARDs (OR, 0.36; 95% CI, 0.1–0.36).

LIMITATIONS OF EXISTING DATA

Although large numbers of patients, prolonged exposure to treatments, and comparative cohorts advance the weight of these data, limited-exposure clinical trial and observational data may be hampered by channeling bias (eg, patients with more severe disease receive aggressive therapies), variable frequency of biologic use in different populations, and the type or quality of the comparator cohorts. Randomized controlled clinical trials provide the most comprehensive data but may also be limited in their application because they are powered to test efficacy and are underpowered to detect rare safety events such as neoplasia. Comparing cancer rates between active drug and placebo may be problematic because of shorter durations of placebo exposure (ie, dropouts, early rescue/exits). Consequently, regulatory agencies opt to compare biologic cancer rates to those seen in the general population, usually with data accrued from an age-matched population studied by the SEER registry. The duration of randomized controlled trials of new drugs may also be insufficient to show the true cancer risk associated with long-term immunosuppression. Open-label extension trials may be long but are biased by the retention of patients who have responded best, often without major safety events.

SUMMARY

The strength of these findings is in the fact that 9 biologics are currently in use and that these have been studied in more than 20,000 patients for the past 10 to 20 years and have been used in more than 3 million patients worldwide. Moreover, greater than 40,000 patients have been enrolled and followed in long-term longitudinal national or regional registries or databases. The reports summarized in this article clearly show that cancers, especially skin cancers, lymphoma, and lung cancers, are increased in patients with RA. Moreover, ample evidence shows that biologic therapies do not alter the risks of many of these cancers, but instead mirror those already seen with the disease. Hence rheumatologists should continue to manage their patients with RA with the best available therapies while the oncologists grapple with cancers if they arise. A great need also exists for consensus between rheumatologists and oncologists about how to manage patients with RA with a cancer concern or diagnosis. Clearly more research is needed to know if continued caution is warranted in patients with a current or past history of melanoma. Lastly, the American College of Rheumatology 2012 guidelines for the management of RA currently recommend rituximab in patients with RA with a treated solid malignancy or NMSC within the past 5 years, those with treated skin melanoma, and those with a treated lymphoproliferative malignancy.[33] This recommendation is without evidence and misleads the prescriber to think that rituximab is a safer drug than the other available biologics. Because cancer risk is more likely to be influenced by uncontrolled inflammation and disease activity, the correct agent to use in the setting of a current or previous malignancy would be the one that will be most apt to control the disease.

REFERENCES

1. Howlader N, Noone AM, Krapcho M, et al, editors. SEER cancer statistics review, 1975-2009 (vintage 2009 populations). Bethesda (MD): National Cancer Institute; 2012. Available at: http://seer.cancer.gov/csr/1975_2009_pops09/. Accessed November 1, 2012.
2. Cush JJ, Dao KH, Kay J. Does rheumatoid arthritis or biologic therapy increase cancer risk? Drug Safety Quarterly 2012;4(2):1–2. Available at: http://www.rheumatology.org/publications/dsq/dsq_2012_08.pdf#toolbar=1. Accessed November 1, 2012.

3. Lopez-Olivo MA, Tayar JH, Martinez-Lopez JA, et al. Risk of malignancies in patients with rheumatoid arthritis treated with biologic therapy: a meta-analysis. JAMA 2012;308:898–908.
4. Smitten AL, Simon TA, Hochberg MC, et al. A meta-analysis of the incidence of malignancy in adult patients with rheumatoid arthritis. Arthritis Res Ther 2008;10:R45.
5. Hellgren K, Smedby KE, Feltelius N, et al. Do rheumatoid arthritis and lymphoma share risk factors?: a comparison of lymphoma and cancer risks before and after diagnosis of rheumatoid arthritis. Arthritis Rheum 2010;62:1252–8.
6. Baecklund E, Iliadou A, Askling J, et al. Association of chronic inflammation, not its treatment, with increased lymphoma risk in rheumatoid arthritis. Arthritis Rheum 2006;54:692–701.
7. Cush JJ, Kavanaugh A. ACR Hotline: FDA Meeting March 2003: Update on the Safety of New Drugs for Rheumatoid Arthritis. American College of Rheumatology Web site. Available at: http://www.rheumatology.org/publications/hotline/0303TNFL.asp. Accessed November 1, 2012.
8. Mariette X, Matucci-Cerinic M, Pavelka K, et al. Malignancies associated with tumour necrosis factor inhibitors in registries and prospective observational studies: a systematic review and meta-analysis. Ann Rheum Dis 2011;70:1895–904.
9. Solomon DH, Mercer E, Kavanaugh A. Observational studies on the risk of cancer associated with tumor necrosis factor inhibitors in rheumatoid arthritis: a review of their methodologies and results. Arthritis Rheum 2012;64:21–32.
10. Singh JA, Wells GA, Christensen R, et al. Adverse effects of biologics: a network meta-analysis and Cochrane overview. Cochrane Database Syst Rev 2011;(2):CD008794.
11. Parakkal D, Sifuentes H, Semer R, et al. Hepatosplenic T-cell lymphoma in patients receiving TNF-α inhibitor therapy: expanding the groups at risk. Eur J Gastroenterol 2011;23:1150–6.
12. Askling J, Fored CM, Brandt L, et al. Risks of solid cancers in patients with rheumatoid arthritis and after treatment with tumour necrosis factor antagonists. Ann Rheum Dis 2005;64:1421–6.
13. Wolfe F, Michaud K. Biologic treatment of rheumatoid arthritis and the risk of malignancy: analyses from a large US observational study. Arthritis Rheum 2007;56:2886–95.
14. Simon TA, Smitten AL, Franklin J, et al. Malignancies in the rheumatoid arthritis abatacept clinical development programme: an epidemiological assessment. Ann Rheum Dis 2009;68:1819–26.
15. Rennard SI, Fogarty C, Kelsen S, et al, COPD Investigators. The safety and efficacy of infliximab in moderate to severe chronic obstructive pulmonary disease. Am J Respir Crit Care Med 2007;175:926–34.
16. Silva F, Seo P, Schroeder DR, et al, Wegener's Granulomatosis Etanercept Trial Research Group. Solid malignancies among etanercept-treated patients with granulomatosis with polyangiitis (Wegener's): long-term followup of a multicenter longitudinal cohort. Arthritis Rheum 2011;63:2495–503.
17. Wenzel SE, Barnes PJ, Bleecker ER, et al, T03 Asthma Investigators. A randomized, double-blind, placebo-controlled study of tumor necrosis factor-alpha blockade in severe persistent asthma. Am J Respir Crit Care Med 2009;179:549–58.
18. Burmester GR, Panaccione R, Gordon KB, et al. Adalimumab: long-term safety in 23 458 patients from global clinical trials in rheumatoid arthritis, juvenile idiopathic arthritis, ankylosing spondylitis, psoriatic arthritis, psoriasis and Crohn's disease. Ann Rheum Dis 2012, in press.
19. Information for Healthcare Professionals: Tumor Necrosis Factor (TNF) Blockers (marketed as Remicade, Enbrel, Humira, Cimzia, and Simponi) FDA ALERT. 2009.

Available at: http://www.fda.gov/Drugs/DrugSafety/PostmarketDrugSafetyInformation forPatientsandProviders/DrugSafetyInformationforHeathcareProfessionals/ucm 174474.htm. Accessed November 1, 2012.

20. Cush JJ, Dao K. FDA Update: TNF inhibitors may increase risk of malignancy in children. Drug Safety Quarterly 2010. Available at: http://www.rheumatology.org/publications/dsq/dsq_2010_01.pdf#toolbar=1. Accessed November 1, 2012.

21. Kemper AR, Van Mater HA, Coeytaux RR, et al. Systematic review of disease-modifying antirheumatic drugs for juvenile idiopathic arthritis. BMC Pediatr 2012;12:29.

22. Bernatsky S, Rosenberg AM, Oen KG, et al. Malignancies in juvenile idiopathic arthritis: a preliminary report. J Rheumatol 2011;38:760–3.

23. Nordstrom BL, Mines D, Gu Y, et al. Risk of malignancy in children with juvenile idiopathic arthritis not treated with biologic agents. Arthritis Care Res 2012;64:1357–64.

24. Simard JF, Neovius M, Hagelberg S, et al. Juvenile idiopathic arthritis and risk of cancer: a nationwide cohort study. Arthritis Rheum 2010;62:3776–82.

25. Beukelman T, Haynes K, Curtis JR, et al. Safety Assessment of Biological Therapeutics Collaboration. Rates of malignancy associated with juvenile idiopathic arthritis and its treatment. Arthritis Rheum 2012;64:1263–71.

26. Watson KD, Dixon WG, Hyrich KL, et al. Influence of anti-TNF therapy and previous malignancy on cancer incidence in patients with rheumatoid arthritis (RA): results from the BSR Biologics Registry. Ann Rheum Dis 2006;65(Suppl II):512.

27. Dixon WG, Watson KD, Lunt M, et al. British Society For Rheumatology Biologics Register Control Centre Consortium; British Society for Rheumatology Biologics Register. Influence of anti-tumor necrosis factor therapy on cancer incidence in patients with rheumatoid arthritis who have had a prior malignancy: results from the British Society for Rheumatology Biologics Register. Arthritis Care Res 2010;62:755–63.

28. Strangfeld A, Hierse F, Rau R, et al. Risk of incident or recurrent malignancies among patients with rheumatoid arthritis exposed to biologic therapy in the German biologics register RABBIT. Arthritis Res Ther 2010;12:R5..

29. Ji J, Liu X, Sundquist K, et al. Survival of cancer in patients with rheumatoid arthritis: a follow-up study in Sweden of patients hospitalized with rheumatoid arthritis 1 year before diagnosis of cancer. Rheumatology 2011;50:1513–8.

30. Franklin J, Lunt M, Bunn D, et al. Influence of inflammatory polyarthritis on cancer incidence and survival: results from a community-based prospective study. Arthritis Rheum 2007;56:790–8.

31. Raaschou P, Simard JF, Neovius M, et al. Anti-Rheumatic Therapy in Sweden Study Group. Does cancer that occurs during or after anti-tumor necrosis factor therapy have a worse prognosis? A national assessment of overall and site-specific cancer survival in rheumatoid arthritis patients treated with biologic agents. Arthritis Rheum 2011;63:1812–22.

32. Carmona L, Descalzo MA, Perez-Pampin E, et al, BIOBADASER and EMECAR Groups. All-cause and cause-specific mortality in rheumatoid arthritis are not greater than expected when treated with tumour necrosis factor antagonists. Ann Rheum Dis 2007;66:880–5.

33. Singh JA, Furst DE, Bharat A, et al. 2012 update of the 2008 American College of Rheumatology recommendations for the use of disease-modifying antirheumatic drugs and biologic agents in the treatment of rheumatoid arthritis. Arthritis Care Res 2012;64:625–39.

Safe Use of Antirheumatic Agents in Patients with Comorbidities

Ashima Makol, MD[1], Kerry Wright, MD[1],
Eric L. Matteson, MD, MPH*

KEYWORDS

- Rheumatoid arthritis • Disease-modifying antirheumatic drugs • Comorbidties
- Adverse drug effects • Treatment

KEY POINTS

- Comorbidities, including cardiovascular (CV) and central nervous system (CNS) disease, chronic kidney disease (CKD), diabetes, and lung disease are common in patients with rheumatoid arthritis (RA).
- Drugs used to treat RA contribute to morbidity in RA, either by causing the comorbid condition or due to heightened risk of toxicity due to the comorbid condition.
- Differentiating drug-related and disease-related morbidity is essential to successful management of risk in patients with RA who have multiple morbidities.

INTRODUCTION

Comorbidities are frequently encountered in patients with RA and, in some situations, as in cases of extra-articular manifestations, are causally related to the disease itself. Management of RA in patients with comorbidities requires a careful balance of the risks and benefits of medications, with consideration of how these have an impact on not only the disease course of RA but also comorbid conditions. Recognition and avoidance of drugs that may exacerbate an underlying comorbid condition are important.

Treatment strategies geared toward more-aggressive treatment early in the disease course and an increase in the number of treatment options, including biologics, influence the occurrence of medication-related side effects and comorbidities. Nonbiologic disease-modifying antirheumatic drugs (DMARDs) have well-recognized side effects, whereas the longer-term impact of biologics is less certain. These factors

Division of Rheumatology, Mayo Clinic College of Medicine, 200 1st Street Southwest, Rochester, MN 55905, USA
[1] Both authors contributed equally toward drafting this article.
* Corresponding author.
E-mail address: matteson.eric@mayo.edu

Rheum Dis Clin N Am 38 (2012) 771–793
http://dx.doi.org/10.1016/j.rdc.2012.08.013
0889-857X/12/$ – see front matter © 2012 Elsevier Inc. All rights reserved.

rheumatic.theclinics.com

increase the challenge of selecting the right medications for the disease and coexistent comorbidities. Physician and patient awareness of possible complications of the medications related to their mechanisms of action and comorbidities, early recognition of adverse events, and prompt discontinuation of any offending agents are important to successful disease management. This review discusses safe use of antirheumatic agents in the setting of comorbid disease in RA.

CARDIOVASCULAR DISEASE AND RHEUMATOID ARTHRITIS TREATMENT

The increased incidence of CV disease (CVD) in patients with RA and higher prevalence of CV risk factors has been well described and is a major contributor to the increased mortality seen in this patient population.

A recent meta-analysis estimated a 50% increase (standardized mortality ratio 1.50; 95% CI, 1.39–1.61) in CV mortality in patients with RA.[1] Heart disease in RA may occur as pericarditis, coronary artery disease, congestive heart failure (CHF), and less commonly amyloidosis, valvular involvement, conduction disturbances, rheumatoid nodules, and coronary arteritis.[2–4]

The increased incidence of CVD seen with RA is in large part related to the underlying disease and inflammatory mechanisms, but the potential for medications to precipitate or exacerbate CVD is well recognized.[5,6]

Patients with RA have higher prevalence of hypertension, obesity, and cigarette smoking as CVD risk factors but no significant difference in the prevalence of diabetes mellitus (DM) or elevated low-density lipoprotein.[7–9] The higher risk of CVD in this population is only partially explained by the presence of traditional CVD risk factors. After controlling for traditional CV risk factors and comorbidities, the risk of CV death was higher among patients with elevated markers of systemic inflammation.[10,11]

Pericarditis

Pericardial disease is the most commonly described cardiac manifestation in RA. Pericardial effusion has been identified in 13% of patients with RA in one series.[12] Evidence of pericardial inflammation has been described in up to 50% of patients in one autopsy series.[13]

Coronary Artery Disease

Accelerated atherogenesis seen with RA is postulated in part due to inflammation, with interaction between immune mechanisms and metabolic factors responsible for the propagation of disease.[14]

Congestive Heart Failure

A population-based retrospective incidence cohort of patients with RA demonstrated a higher incidence of CHF among patients with RA (rate ratio [RR] 1.7; 95% CI, 1.3–2.1). RA conferred a significant excess risk of CHF (hazard ratio [HR] 1.87; 95% CI, 1.47–2.39) after adjusting for demographics, ischemic heart disease, and CVD risk factors.[11] CHF has been shown a greater contributor to excess mortality than ischemic heart disease as a result of the increase in incidence rather than a worse prognosis for CHF in patients with RA.[15]

Noncardiac Vascular Disease

A population-based incidence cohort study of patients with RA did not show an increase in the incidence of peripheral arterial or cerebrovascular disease but reported a higher incidence of venous thromboembolism.[16] Recent studies have suggested an increased incidence of atrial fibrillation in patients with RA with an adjusted incidence RR of 1.41 (95% CI, 1.31–1.51).[17]

Drug Safety and Cardiovascular Disease in Rheumatoid Arthritis

The safety of drugs used in RA is summarized here and in **Table 1**.

Biologics

Tumor necrosis factor α inhibitors Tumor necrosis factor α (TNF-α) inhibition was considered a potential target for therapy for CHF; however, several trials of TNF blockers, principally infliximab, for management of CHF failed to show any treatment benefits and suggested potential harm.[18,19] There was a trend toward a worse outcome in patients with nonischemic heart disease and in those less than 65 years of age.[20] At least one study comparing patients treated with anti-TNF inhibitors to patients on conventional DMARDs over a 5-year study period did not reveal an increase in all-cause mortality or CVD mortality.[21]

Data regarding outcomes in patients with RA are largely derived from observational cohorts and long-term extension studies of the TNF inhibitors and have not been as conclusive as the data obtained from studies of patients without RA. Analysis of data from a German prospective observational cohort study (RABBIT) revealed, after adjustment for traditional CV risk factors, that the risk of developing heart failure was higher in patients with evidence of greater disease activity (HR 1.47; 95% CI, 1.07–2.02; P = 0.019). A smaller study found that the risk of new or worsening heart failure was not significantly greater in patients treated with anti-TNF agents.[16]

The impact of treatment with TNF inhibitors on the risk of CHF was examined in an observational cohort of 13,171 patients with RA. CHF was reported in 461 cases, including 42 incident cases, 24 of which occurred in patients without pre-existing CVD.[22] Among all cases of CHF (both prevalent and incident), patients receiving

Table 1
Cardiac safety of drugs in rheumatoid arthritis

Disease-Modifying Antirheumatic Drugs	
1. HCQ	Overall safe Rare case reports of cardiomyopathy

2. Other Non-Biologics
     methotrexate
     Leflunomide
     Sulfasalazine
	Overall safe
	Potential reduction in CV mortality

Glucocorticoids	Increased risk of MI Minimize dose and duration of use
Biologic Response Modifiers	

1. Anti-TNF agents
     (etanercept, infliximab adalimumab,
     golimumab, and certolizumab)
	Worsening heart failure
	• Avoid in patients with heart failure: NYHA
	  class III or greater and left ventricular ejection
	  fraction <50%
	• Potential benefit in patients with CAD

2. Tocilizumab	Overall safe
3. Abatacept	No increase in risk of CV events reported
4. Rituximab	
NSAIDs	Increased risk of CV events • Avoid in patients with a history of CV disease • Minimize dose and duration of exposure

anti-TNF therapy were less likely to have CHF than were those not receiving anti-TNF treatment. The frequency of CHF was 1.2% lower in anti-TNF–treated patients. It is likely that the number of patients at risk for CHF was low in this observational cohort because of the warnings against use of infliximab in patients with heart failure.[22]

The American College of Rheumatology recommends that in patients with RA with CHF that is New York Heart Association (NYHA) class III or IV and an ejection fraction of 50% or less that an anti-TNF biologic not be used.[23]

The results from one observational study (CORRONA registry) indicated a lower risk for a composite outcome of nonfatal myocardial infarction (MI), transient ischemic attack, or stroke and CV-related death in patients treated with TNF antagonists (HR 0.39; 95% CI, 0.19–0.82) compared with users of nonbiologic DMARDs.[24] A prospective observational study using the British Society for Rheumatology Biologics Register (BSRBR) showed a decrease in the incidence of MI in the subset of patients with a response to anti–TNF-α treatment within 6 months (adjusted incidence ratio of 0.36; 95% CI, 0.19–0.69) in comparison with nonresponders.[25]

A recent meta-analysis of randomized controlled trials showed a trend toward reduction in risk of events although this failed to achieve statistical significance.[26] The risk of MI in patients treated with a TNF inhibitor does not seem to be increased and studies suggest potential benefit.

Rituximab In 49 patients with RA treated with rituximab, one study suggested a beneficial effect with a less atherogenic cholesterol profile at 6 months in patients who responded to treatment.[27] The changes in lipid levels observed were small and it is unclear how this will have an impact on atherosclerotic risk in the long term. Long-term safety data of 2578 patients with 5013 patient-years of follow-up have not demonstrated any increase in the risk of CV events in comparison with placebo.[28]

Abatacept Abatacept has also been shown to have a beneficial effect on lipid profile after 24 weeks of treatment.[29] A systematic review of randomized controlled trials of abatacept, including long-term extension studies for treatment of RA, did not demonstrate an increased risk of CV events.[30]

Tocilizumab High circulating levels of interleukin (IL)-6 have been associated with increased risk of coronary artery disease. On the basis of genetic evidence in humans, it has been postulated that IL-6 blockade could serve as a potential therapeutic target in prevention of coronary artery disease (CAD).[31]

Lipid abnormalities have been reported as an adverse effect in the clinical trials of tocilizumab (TCZ) with increases in total cholesterol, high-density lipoprotein cholesterol, and triglyceride levels.[32–34] Long-term extension studies have not reported an increase in the risk of CV events.[35] Pooled long-term data from clinical trials showed that the rates of MI and stroke were consistent with those expected for patients with RA and remained stable.[36]

Anakinra A randomized placebo-controlled trial of anakinra use in patients with comorbid disease, including prior history of a CV event, did not demonstrate any increase in the rate of CV events at 6 months.[37]

Nonbiologic DMARDs

Methotrexate Methotrexate (MTX) has been the most studied, but there has been suggestion that other DMARDs may also be associated with a reduced risk of CV disease although the data have not been as conclusive. A nested case-control study of patients with RA with no prior history of CHF demonstrated a 30% risk reduction for CHF hospitalization with use of any DMARD.[38]

The risk of acute MI associated with use of DMARDs was significantly lower among patients currently on a DMARD (adjusted RR 0.80; 95% CI, 0.65–0.98) compared with age-matched and gender-matched controls, and was significant for MTX, leflunomide, and other traditional DMARDs (including hydroxychloroquine [HCQ]) and sulfasalazine [SSZ]).[39] A large cross-sectional international study of 4363 patients with RA looked at hospitalization with MI in patients treated with DMARDs based on years of exposure to the medications. In addition to an 18% reduction in the risk of MI in patients treated with MTX for 1 year, longer use of leflunomide and SSZ was also associated with a reduction in the risk of MI (adjusted HR: SSZ 0.82 [0.69–0.98] and leflunomide 0.52 [0.26–1.06]) even after adjusting for disease severity and CV risk factors.[40]

All-cause mortality may be reduced by as much as 60% and CV mortality reduced by as much as 70% in patients with RA treated with MTX.[41–44]

Antimalarials A reversible drug-induced cardiomyopathy has been reported rarely with use of HCQ and chloroquine.[15,45] In a nested case-control study of patients with RA, HCQ was not associated with an increase in CV events.[46] There is no contraindication for use of antimalarials in patients with heart failure because cardiomyopathy is rare.

Glucocorticoids

Use of prednisone has been associated with a dose-dependent increase in the risk of MI of up to 50%.[24,39,46] Additional studies have suggested that the higher risk of CV events occurs in patients with steroid exposure in a dose-dependent manner, especially in rheumatoid factor–positive patients.[47–49]

Nonsteroidal anti-inflammatory drugs

Patients treated with nonsteroidal anti-inflammatory drugs (NSAIDs), including cyclooxygenase (COX) II inhibitors, are at higher risk of heart failure, especially those with a pre-existing diagnosis of heart failure in a dose-dependent manner.[50–52]

Both nonselective NSAIDs and COX-2 inhibitors are associated with an increase in blood pressure and sodium and water retention, which are contributors to the risk of CHF exacerbation.[50,53,54]

A meta-analysis of large-scale, randomized controlled trials comparing different NSAIDs against each other or placebo demonstrated the highest risk of stroke with ibuprofen use (HR 3.36; 95% CI, 1.00–11.6). Diclofenac was found associated with one of the highest risks of death (HR 3.98; 95% CI, 1.48–12.7). Of the NSAIDs investigated, naproxen was associated with the least harm.[55]

Key Points

- TNF inhibitors should be avoided in patients with heart failure (NYHA class III or IV) or a left ventricular ejection fraction of <50%.
- MTX use may be associated with a lower risk of CV mortality.
- Use of NSAIDs in patients with a history of CV disease should be avoided if at all possible. If used, however, they should be at the lowest dose and for the shortest duration. Both selective and nonselective NSAIDs are associated with increased risk but the risk may be somewhat less with use of naproxen
- Use of glucocorticoids is associated with a higher risk of MI.

CENTRAL NERVOUS SYSTEM DISEASE AND RHEUMATOID ARTHRITIS TREATMENT

CNS disease may be seen as an extra-articular manifestation of RA with the most common manifestation cervical myelopathy as a result of atlantoaxial subluxation. Prior estimates of the prevalence of cervical spine involvement have been as high as 86% with neurologic deficits and cervical myelopathy reported less frequently.[56] CNS vasculitis occurring with RA is rare.[57,58] Rarely, pachymeningitis or leptomeningitis, vasculitis, and intracranial rheumatoid nodules have been reported in patients with severe long-standing disease.[59]

Demyelinating Disease

Demyelinating disease occurring with RA has become more of a concern recently with use of TNF inhibitors. There is no clear association between RA and demyelinating disease, including multiple sclerosis.[60–62]

Safety of Biologics Used to Treat Rheumatoid Arthritis in CNS Disease

Demyelinating disease has been described as an adverse side effect associated with use of TNF inhibitors. A pharmacologic database-derived cohort of 104,598 RA patients with no prior history of a confirmed demyelinating event recorded 253 newly confirmed demyelinating events (209 cases of multiple sclerosis and 44 cases of optic neuritis) during an average follow-up of 1.9 person-years. Patients with a prior suspected demyelination event prior to start of treatment had the highest risk of an event with use of anakinra (RR 2.74; 95% CI, 1.59–4.74).[60]

Among patients with no suspected demyelination prior to entry, the adjusted RR for an event after exposure remained, but to a lesser extent (RR 1.31; 0.68–2.50), and was not much higher compared with other nonbiologic DMARDs: MTX (1.09; 0.63–1.89]), leflunomide (1.52; 0.71–3.28), and antimalarials (1.16; 0.64–2.09).[60] Review of Food and Drug Administration adverse events reporting identified 19 patients who had neurologic events after TNF administration (17 patients with etanercept and 2 after infliximab). In cases where the TNF inhibitor was discontinued, patients had partial or complete resolution of symptoms with one patient having improvement and recurrence with rechallenge. Four patients had prior history of multiple sclerosis or multiple sclerosis–like syndromes.[63]

Isolated optic neuritis was reported in a case series of 15 patients on anti-TNF agents, including 8 on infliximab, 5 on etanercept, and 2 on adalimumab. The optic neuritis occurred at a median of 7.5 months (range 2 months to 1.5 years) with the majority of patients (11) having complete or partial resolution with treatment with prednisone. Anti–TNF-α treatment was continued in 2 patients, 1 experiencing partial resolution and the other having ongoing symptoms.[64]

The impact of TCZ, rituximab, and abatacept on demyelinating disease is not known.

Key Points

- Use of a TNF inhibitor should be avoided in patients with history of multiple sclerosis or patients with an event suggestive of demyelinating disease.

- In patients treated with a TNF inhibitor who develop neurologic symptoms, early recognition, discontinuation of the agent, and further evaluation are important.

DIABETES MELLITUS AND RHEUMATOID ARTHRITIS TREATMENT

Evidence from population-based cohort studies has not suggested an increase in the prevalence of DM among patients with RA compared with non-RA subjects.[10,65,66] It is possible that treatment strategies geared at controlling inflammation may improve insulin sensitivity, glycemic control, and glucose metabolism.[67]

Nonsteroidal Anti-inflammatory Drugs

Larger than conventional doses of NSAIDs have been associated with hypoglycemia but at usual doses any hypoglycemic effect is usually minimal.[68] Avoidance of use of NSAIDs in patients with DM is recommended because of the associated risk of renal disease.

Glucocorticoids

Glucocorticoid use is known to be associated with a risk of hyperglycemia, in particular when used at higher doses. Among nondiabetic patients with RA treated with steroids, previous exposure to oral prednisone or high doses of pulsed glucocorticoids are associated with decreased insulin sensitivity.[69] Reports of patients with RA treated over a 25-year period with low doses of prednisone (5 mg/d or less) did not suggest an increase in the risk of DM.[70]

Patients with RA with pre-existing DM treated with steroids had worsening of their DM control 3 to 6 months after initiation of corticosteroid therapy.[71]

Patients starting on corticosteroids for long-term treatment should have a baseline fasting blood glucose measurement. Close glucose monitoring is important in patients with a pre-existing diagnosis of DM.

Nonbiologic DMARDS

HCQ use by nondiabetic women with RA is associated with lower fasting glucose levels.[72] Among patients with RA and DM, HCQ use is associated with a 0.54% greater reduction in hemogloblin (Hb) A_{1c} than use of MTX.[73]

SSZ seems to have modest glucose-lowering properties. A hypoglycemic effect is reported with doses as a low as 1 g/d but was more frequent with higher doses.[74] There have been no reports of DMARDS resulting in poor glycemic control in patients with DM.

Biologics

TNF-α inhibitors

A retrospective cohort study of patients with either RA or psoriasis with no prior history of DM followed for a mean duration of 5.8 months reported that patients started on treatment with anti-TNF agents or HCQ had a lower rate of DM.[24] Use of both infliximab and etanercept has been associated with improved insulin resistance in nondiabetic patients with RA. This effect was not seen with adalimumab although the number of patients was small and exposure short.[67] Review of 1587 incident cases of nondiabetic RA revealed that use of TNF inhibitors was associated with a 51% reduction in the incidence of DM, after adjusting for covariates (including glucocorticoid use, body mass index, and erythrocyte sedimentation rate).[67]

There are no randomized controlled trials of TNF inhibitors examining their impact on glycemic control in patients with DM but animal studies and retrospective studies suggest a possible benefit.[75,76] Athough patients with DM are at higher risk of infection, this risk does not seem elevated among diabetic patients treated with a TNF inhibitor who developed an infection.[77]

Anakinra

A double-blind, parallel-group, placebo-controlled trial of 70 patients with established type 2 DM treated with either anakinra (100 mg daily) or placebo for 13 weeks showed that among the group of patients receiving anakinra the HbA_{1c} was 0.46% lower than in the placebo group with no reports of symptomatic hypoglycemia.[78]

Tocilizumab

IL-6 has been found increased in patients with DM, and inhibition of IL-6 signaling with TCZ in 11 patients with RA was associated with improvement in insulin sensitivity in one study.[79]

LUNG DISEASE AND RHEUMATOID ARTHRITIS TREATMENT

Comorbid pulmonary disease is common in RA patients. It may be prevalent prior to RA onset and affect choice of initial therapy or develop during the course of disease as an extra-articular complication and may be severe enough to merit precedence over treatment of articular disease. Certain DMARDs and biologics are associated with risk of drug-induced lung injury, posing a contraindication to their use in patients with pre-existent lung disease. Several features of pulmonary involvement in RA have been described (**Box 1**), including nodulosis, pleural involvement, interstitial lung disease (ILD), obstructive airway disease, and, rarely, vasculitis.

Key Points

- With the exception of use of glucocorticoids, medications used to manage RA, including traditional and biologic DMARDs, do not seem to increase the risk of development of DM or worsening glycemic control among patients with a diagnosis of DM.
- Disease-modifying therapies may potentially improve glycemic control.
- Use of disease-modifying therapies may be associated with a reduction in the incidence of DM among patients with RA.

Interstitial Lung Disease in Rheumatoid Arthritis

Prevalence of ILD in RA ranges from as high as 8.2% in recent-onset RA to a cumulative prevalence of 19% to 44%[80–84] depending on the study and modality used to make the diagnosis (chest radiograph, high-resolution CT, spirometry, or lung biopsy). It has a diversity of histopathologic patterns with the predominant picture being usual interstitial pneumonia (33%), nonspecific interstitial pneumonia (33%), and bronchiolitis obliterans organizing pneumonia (11%).[85] The risk of death for RA patients with ILD is 3 times higher than in RA patients without ILD (HR 2.86; 95% CI, 1.98–4.12) and median survival after ILD diagnosis is only 2.6 years. ILD contributes approximately 13% to the excess mortality of RA patients compared with the general population.[86]

Treatment of RA-ILD remains somewhat empiric. High daily dose of corticosteroids effectively suppresses a rapidly progressive disease process but reactivation often occurs with tapering the dose. Immunosuppressive agents, in particular azathioprine with or without N-acetylcysteine, must be considered along with prednisone in these patients, given the reported clinical efficacy in idiopathic pulmonary fibrosis.[87] Other treatments include mycophenolate mofetil,[88] rituximab,[89] and cyclophosphamide.

Pulmonary infections are reported a major cause of death in RA.[90] Bacterial (including typical and atypical mycobacteria, legionella, and listeria) and fungal

Box 1
Pulmonary involvement in rheumatoid arthritis
Pleural disease
1. Pleurisy
2. Pleural effusion
3. Empyema
4. Pneumothorax
Rheumatoid nodules (lung parenchyma)
1. Caplan syndrome (nodules with pneumoconiosis)
Interstitial lung disease
1. Nonspecific interstitial pneumonia
2. Usual interstitial pneumonia
3. Bronchiolitis obliterans organizing pneumonia
4. Lymphocytic interstitial pneumonia
Obstructive airway disease
1. Obliterative bronchiolitis
2. Bronchiectasis
Pulmonary vasculitis
Drug-induced lung disease
1. Methotrexate
2. Sulfasalazine
3. Leflunomide
4. Anti-TNF agents

pneumonias are common, can be recurrent, and often lead to bronchiectasis. They may arise de novo, but the risk is increased several-fold by the degree of immunosuppression and coexistent ILD. The risk of pulmonary infections is increased with most DMARDs but HCQ and SSZ seem safe in the authors' experience. Most biologic response modifiers carry a black box warning for increased risk of opportunistic infections, some leading to hospitalization or death. High-dose corticosteroid use is a major risk factor for *Pneumocystis jiroveci* pneumonia, and the authors recommend prophylaxis for *Pneumocystis jiroveci* pneumonia in all patients on corticosteroids at a dose of greater than 20-mg prednisone equivalent.

Drug-Induced Lung Injury in Rheumatoid Arthritis

Drug-induced pulmonary toxicity clinically presents with unexplained fever, cough, dyspnea, hypoxemia, and infiltrates on chest radiograph without microbiologic evidence of infection on cultures. Issues in drug safety and lung disease in RA are summarized in **Table 2**.

Nonbiologic DMARDs

Methotrexate Historically, rapidly progressive interstitial pneumonitis has been the most serious complication associated with MTX use,[91] with a reported frequency of

Table 2
Pulmonary safety of drug treatment in rheumatoid arthritis

Disease-Modifying Antirheumatic Drugs	
1. Hydroxychloroquine	No safety concerns
2. Methotrexate	MTX-induced pneumonitis
	• Avoid in moderate to advanced ILD
	• Use with caution in patients with interstitial changes on chest radiography or restrictive changes on PFT
	• Avoid use in combination with anti-TNF agents in patients with ILD
3. Leflunomide	Pneumonitis in Japanese and Koreans
4. Sulfasalazine	Hypersensitivity pneumonitis to the sulfapyridine moiety, rare
	Reversible after discontinuing the drug
5. Intramuscular gold	Constrictive bronchiolitis and obstructive airway
6. D-Penicillamine	disease
7. Azathioprine	Safe from pulmonary standpoint
8. Mycophenolate mofetil	Often used for treatment of RA-ILD
9. Cyclophosphamide	

Biologic Response Modifiers	
1. Anti-TNF agents (etanercept, infliximab, and adalimumab)	May induce or exacerbate ILD
	May potentiate pulmonary toxicity of MTX
2. Newer anti-TNF agents (golimumab, certolizumab)	Rare reports of fibrosing alveolitis and noninfectious pneumonitis
3. Tocilizumab	Overall safe
	Rare reports of ILD and noninfectious pneumonitis
4. Abatacept	Safe in ILD
	Exacerbation of obstructive lung disease
	Avoid in COPD
5. Rituximab	Reports of ILD and deaths in patients with hematologic malignancy
	• Similar events rare in RA patients
	• Use with caution

3% to as high as 18%.[92,93] Although there is no universally accepted definition for MTX-induced pneumonitis, it is believed an acute to subacute hypersensitivity reaction, often leading to rapidly progressive dyspnea, acute respiratory failure, and, in rare cases, death.[94] It is neither duration-limited nor dose-related and has been reported at doses as low as 12.5 mg/wk.[95–97]

It is difficult to predict the development of this uncommon complication, but patients with baseline pulmonary function abnormalities from ILD[92,97] or pre-existing lung disease[95] are believed at greatest risk. Reduced pulmonary reserve portends a worse prognosis.[25] Advanced age, pre-existing interstitial abnormalities, and previous adverse reactions to DMARDs may be associated with MTX pneumonitis.[98] A few studies have shown male gender,[97] renal insufficiency,[99] and concurrent use of salicylates[100] to predispose to MTX pneumonitis, but others have not corroborated their results.

In view of these concerns, the American College of Physicians Health and Public Policy Committee's guidelines list pre-existing lung disease as an absolute contraindication for MTX use in RA patients.[99] Given the high efficacy of MTX as a DMARD and rarity of MTX-induced pneumonitis, however, it is considered a contraindication by most clinicians. It is prudent to consider a baseline chest radiograph and/or pulmonary function tests (PFTs) to assess for pre-existing lung disease in all patients in whom treatment with MTX is contemplated and to discuss the risks and benefits with patients. It may be best to monitor patients with pre-existing lung disease or interstitial changes on radiographs closely for pulmonary side effects. Although reintroduction of MTX after MTX pneumonitis is not always followed by pulmonary toxicity,[101,102] this must be done with caution.

Other DMARDs There are no reports of pulmonary toxicity with HCQ. Leflunomide is also safe from a pulmonary standpoint but has rarely been reported to cause pneumonitis. Reports are more frequent among Korean and Japanese patients[103] but patients with a history of MTX pneumonitis are also at risk of developing pneumonitis with leflunomide.[89]

Pulmonary toxicity due to SSZ was reported in a series of 50 cases, only 6 of which were using it for RA.[104] Toxicity is believed a hypersensitivity reaction mediated by the sulfapyridine moiety. Discontinuation of SSZ led to resolution of symptoms in 90% of the cases after an average of 6.5 weeks, whereas 20 patients were simultaneously treated with addition of corticosteroids. There were 5 fatalities, all among patients on high-dose SSZ (mean dose 3.6 g) for inflammatory bowel disease. Overall, the incidence of pulmonary toxicity with SSZ is low and it reverses with prompt discontinuation of the drug.

Biologics
Anti-TNF agents Anti-TNF agents have been reported to induce or exacerbate ILD in RA patients.[105] Whether this is related to the TNF antagonist itself or the often concomitantly administered MTX has been difficult to tease out. These agents are thought to shift the systemic and/or pulmonary environment toward anti-inflammatory cytokines, such as transforming growth factor $\beta1$, which in turn contribute to a profibrotic state.[106] By promoting deficient apoptosis of infiltrating inflammatory cells and enhancing release of macrophage-derived proteolytic enzymes, these drugs may further enhance the potential pulmonary toxicity of MTX.

Perez-Alvarez and colleagues[105] reported 122 cases of new-onset or exacerbation of ILD secondary to biologics as part of the BIOGEAS project, a multicenter study dedicated to collecting data on the use of biologic agents in patients with systemic autoimmune diseases. Among these, etanercept was the offending drug in 58 cases and infliximab in 56 cases; 89% of the cases received the drugs for RA. Two-thirds of the patients had received or were receiving MTX. ILD was reported a mean of 26 weeks after anti-TNF initiation and was confirmed by pulmonary biopsy in 26 cases. Treatment included withdrawal of the biologic in all but 1 patient; 21 cases had complete resolution and 13 had partial resolution but no improvement was noted in 18 patients. There were 15 deaths during follow-up, the majority within the first 5 weeks after initiating the biologic. Those patients who died were more likely to be aged greater than 65 years (67% vs 33%, $P = .04$), had later onset of ILD (46 weeks vs 15 weeks, $P = .006$), were more likely to have had a prior diagnosis of ILD (67% vs 29%, $P = .025$), and received immunosuppressive drugs more frequently (33% vs 8%, $P = .04$).

Dixon and colleagues[107] compared 10,649 RA patients treated with anti-TNF therapy in the BSRBR to 3464 RA patients treated with nonbiologic DMARDs and found a higher prevalence of physician-reported ILD in the former group, 299 cases versus 68 cases (2.8% vs 1.9%, $P = .006$, OR 1.44). The BSRBR data also showed that patients with pre-existing pulmonary disease (n = 184) had a 6-fold higher mortality rate when treated with anti-TNF agents than patients without pulmonary disease (n = 6061) (90 vs 14 per 1000 person-years of follow-up).

Tocilizumab A systematic literature review of TCZ, including 3 controlled trials, reported 6 adverse events among 589 patients (1%) that included new-onset ILD, *idiopathic pulmonary fibrosis*, allergic pneumonitis, and 3 cases of culture-negative pneumonia; 4 of them were concomitantly on MTX.[38] In addition, a case of fatal exacerbation of RA-associated ILD has also been reported with TCZ alone.[108] Storage and colleagues[109] reviewed safety data from all published TCZ trials and found 170 minor pulmonary adverse effects (noninfectious) in the treatment group versus 70 in the placebo group but no cases of ILD or parenchymal lung disease were noted.

Abatacept Abatacept is associated with exacerbation of chronic obstructive pulmonary disease and should be avoided in patients with moderate to severe obstructive airway disease.[110,111]

Rituximab The pulmonary safety of rituximab is uncertain. Among more than 100,000 patients (with no evidence of ILD at baseline) treated with high-dose rituximab for lymphoma or other hematologic malignancies over a decade, a total of 45 cases of ILD and 8 deaths were reported.[112,113] Alternatively, experience from the Dose-Ranging Assessment: International Clinical Evaluation of Rituximab in Rheumatoid Arthritis trial demonstrated only 1 case of ILD among 316 patients (0.32%), and that patient was on concomitant MTX treatment.[114] An open-label study of the efficacy of rituximab in RA-related ILD was inconclusive.[115]

Key Points

- Chronic lung disease, especially ILD, is an independent factor associated with increased mortality in RA.
- Screening for and identifying comorbid lung disease early in the course of a patient's disease may help in identifying appropriate DMARD regimens with least risk of drug-induced pulmonary toxicity. This may be accomplished with a baseline chest radiograph and/or PFT, which also help for future comparison and may help distinguish RA-ILD from drug-induced lung injury.
- MTX should be used with caution in patients with pre-existent interstitial changes on chest radiograph or restrictive changes on PFT.
- MTX alone and its combination with anti-TNF agents should be avoided in patients with moderate to severe ILD.

KIDNEY DISEASE AND RHEUMATOID ARTHRITIS TREATMENT

Renal dysfunction may be prevalent in RA but often goes unrecognized either due a slow rate of progression or inadequacy of the serum creatinine level to be a good representation of decline in renal function.[116]

Renal Dysfunction in Rheumatoid Arthritis

RA preferentially affects joints and soft tissues, but the inflammatory process can commonly extend to involve solid organs, including, on rare occasion, the kidney (**Box 2**). Boers[117] hypothesized the presence of a nonspecific subclinical nephropathy, characterized by nephrosclerosis and mesangial hypercellularity, from cumulative minor insults caused by the disease and its treatment, which makes RA patients sensitive to other renal insults and accounts for the high prevalence of renal failure at death.

Box 2
Classification of renal dysfunction in rheumatoid arthritis

1. Renal disorders from RA and its complications

   a. Rheumatoid nephropathy

   b. AA amyloidosis

   c. Renal vasculitis

   d. Glomerulonephritis

2. Drug-induced renal disorders

   a. NSAIDS

      i. Analgesic nephropathy with papillary necrosis

      ii. Acute interstitial nephritis

      iii. Chronic interstitial nephritis

   b. Gold and ᴅ-penicillamine

      i. Membranous glomerulonephritis

      ii. Nephrotic syndrome

   c. Cyclosporin A

      i. Obliterative arteriolopathy and tubular atrophy with scarring

3. Comorbid chronic renal dysfunction from

   a. Hypertension

   b. Diabetes mellitus

   c. Sjögren syndrome

      i. Interstitial nephritis and distal renal tubular acidosis

---

Rarely, rheumatoid vasculitis with renal involvement occurs as a severe complication of longstanding, nodular, erosive RA with necrotizing immune complex–mediated rapidly progressing GN with extracapillary proliferation, and that requires intense immunosuppression.[118,119]

Longstanding chronic inflammation from poorly controlled RA can also result in deposition of inert fibrillar material, consisting of serum amyloid A protein in the kidneys causing renal AA amyloidosis (secondary amyloidosis), a rare yet serious and potentially life-threatening disorder. This complication has become rare in the modern era of RA treatment.[55–57] In addition, toxicity of DMARDs can affect the kidney.

Mortality Associated with Renal Dysfunction in Rheumatoid Arthritis

Although given little attention during the lifetime of a patient with RA, regardless of the cause, concurrent renal disease has been shown a predictor of mortality in these patients. Mortality from renal disease has been seen to range between 10% and 34% in RA.[120,121] A prospective study comparing 1000 RA cases with an equal number of age-matched and gender-matched controls over 10 years found 20% of deaths attributed to renal disease in the cases compared with only 1% among controls.[120] A population-based study from Finland determined an HR for mortality from nephropathy of 1.78.[122]

Clinical Presentation of Renal Dysfunction in Rheumatoid Arthritis

In a prospective study of 235 patients with early RA, 7% of patients developed persistent proteinuria and 6% elevated serum creatinine with or without proteinuria during a 42-month observation period.[123] These were mostly treatment related and reversed after discontinuation of the offending drug. D-penicillamine and gold (but not MTX) were most often associated with proteinuria. In the Methotrexate and Renal Insufficiency (MATRIX) study and elevated serum creatinine values were found in 19% of prevalent RA patients.[124] Among these, 20% were in stage 2 and 15% were in stage 3 of chronic kidney disease (CKD). Proteinuria, hematuria, and leukocyturia were observed in 16%, 17%, and 20% of the patients, respectively, but the cause of renal pathology was not determined in this study.[124]

Histopathology of Renal Dysfunction in Rheumatoid Arthritis

Retrospective analysis of renal biopsies performed on specimens from 110 RA patients with clinical renal disease attributed to antirheumatic therapy or RA itself was reported by Helin and colleagues.[125] All patients presented with isolated hematuria, isolated proteinuria, both, or acute renal failure. The most common histopathological finding was mesangial glomerulonephritis (GN) in 36% (n = 40), followed by amyloidosis (30%, n = 33) and membranous GN (17%, n = 19). Focal proliferative GN (4%, n = 4), minimal change nephropathy (3%, n = 3), and acute interstitial nephritis (1%, n = 1) were less common. Amyloidosis was the most frequent finding in those with nephrotic syndrome. In patients with isolated proteinuria, amyloidosis, membranous GN, and mesangial GN were equally common.[125] Membranous GN was closely related to gold or D-penicillamine therapy, whereas mesangial GN was probably related to RA itself. Necrotizing vasculitis with rapidly progressive GN and extracapillary proliferation was rare and noted in only 2 patients. A similar spectrum of lesions was reported from other studies as well.[126–128] Drug-induced proteinuria regressed in most patients and was associated with a good prognosis. Alternatively, proteinuria from amyloidosis is often progressive and associated with high mortality rates.

Nephrotoxicity of Drug Treatment in Rheumatoid Arthritis

NSAIDS

Chronic use of NSAIDS was once implicated in causing analgesic-induced nephropathy characterized by papillary necrosis and interstitial nephritis. Chronic interstitial nephritis has been reported in RA patients with analgesic abuse but is uncommon[129] if the use of NSAIDS is intermittent, under medical supervision, and with a single agent. NSAIDs can rarely induce an acute interstitial nephritis with proteinuria, eosinophilia, and eosinophiluria, an allergic phenomenon that is reversible after discontinuing the drug. NSAIDs (including COX-2 inhibitors) can cause acute deterioration of renal function, which is more common particularly in elderly, CKD patients, CHF patients, and states of volume depletion, because renal blood flow is dependent on renal prostaglandin synthesis.[130,131] Glucocorticoids, acetaminophen, or opioids are a suitable alternative to replace NSAIDs in RA patients with CKD.

Nonbiologic DMARDS

Gold and D-penicillamine The 2 most common DMARDS associated with nephrotoxicity are gold (oral and injectable) and D-penicillamine, both rarely used now.

Cyclosporin A Cyclosporin A renal toxicity manifests primarily as a significant increase in serum creatinine level.[132] This is mediated via its vasoconstrictive effect on the afferent and efferent glomerular arterioles, leading to a reduction in renal blood flow and creatinine clearance.[133] Long-term use can cause obliterative arteriolopathy, ischemic scarring, tubular atrophy, and progressive loss of renal function.[117] Risk factors include high dose, advanced age, and pre-existing CKD.[134] Abnormalities of renal function improved with discontinuing or lowering the dose of cyclosporine.

Use of cyclosporine hence is contraindicated in RA patients with renal dysfunction in accordance with consensus guidelines.[135] Its use is recommended with caution in patients older than 65 years of age, due to a higher risk of renal dysfunction, and among patients on drugs that may independently promote renal dysfunction (like NSAIDS).[135]

Methotrexate MTX is primarily excreted via the kidneys (approximately 90%). Although considered minimally nephrotoxic, several studies have confirmed an associated with subtle changes in renal function with the most consistent association decrease in creatinine clearance.[136,137] Its own clearance from the body may be affected with MTX toxicity occurring with worsening CKD. Pooled results from 11 trials involving 496 patients showed that patients with compromised renal function had the highest overall rates of MTX toxicity with 4 times higher odds of severe toxicity, including severe respiratory problems, compared with patients with normal creatinine clearance.[138] Dose reduction of MTX is prudent in CKD patients and should generally be avoided in advanced CKD patients.

Antimalarials Antimalarials have a generally safe renal profile. In one study,[139] 118 patients were noted to have a greater than 10% decline in their creatinine clearance after initiating antimalarials—55% patients on chloroquine compared with 15% with HCQ. Age was found a strong independent predictor of nephrotoxicity. Up to 40% of HCQ is excreted unchanged in urine. Dose adjustment seems prudent in patients with abnormal renal function.[140]

Other DMARDs SSZ seems generally safe from a renal standpoint.[141] Because of partial excretion of its metabolites by the kidneys, dose reductions have been proposed at a glomerular filtration rate less than 50 mL/min.[132] Similarly, large clinical trials of leflunomide[142,143] and azathioprine[144,145] have not demonstrated any sign of renal toxicity. Leflunomide, however, often increases blood pressure, which adds blood pressure monitoring and blood pressure control (<130/80 mm Hg) to the responsibilities of rheumatologists. Leflunomide is predominantly excreted in bile and clearance is not affected by renal function. No dose change is necessary in patients on hemodialysis.[146]

Biologics

Anti-TNF agents are regarded as safe to use from the renal standpoint and seem safe in patients on renal dialysis.[94] These are hydrolyzed at the level of lysosomes and no unchanged drug is excreted in the urine.[94]

Key Points

- Patients with RA must be routinely monitored by blood (serum creatinine and estimated glomerular filtration rate) and urinary parameters (urinalysis with microscopy) for concomitant CKD, which can be either a manifestation of their RA or a side effect of DMARD therapy or another disease process.

- Modification of RA therapy may be required because of kidney disease.

There is a dearth of data on renal safety of other biologics. Abatacept has not been studied in patients with renal impairment. Rituximab demonstrated no change in pharmacokinetics when used in lymphoma patients on hemodialysis and is believed safe in patients with renal insufficiency.[147] TCZ does not need dose adjustment in mild renal insufficiency but has not been studied in moderate to severe renal insufficiency.

REFERENCES

1. Avina-Zubieta JA, Choi HK, Sadatsafavi M, et al. Risk of cardiovascular mortality in patients with rheumatoid arthritis: a meta-analysis of observational studies. Arthritis Rheum 2008;59(12):1690–7.
2. Cruickshank B. The arteritis of rheumatoid arthritis. Ann Rheum Dis 1954;13(2): 136–46.
3. Kitas G, Banks MJ, Bacon PA. Cardiac involvement in rheumatoid disease. Clin Med 2001;1(1):18–21.
4. Wislowska M, Sypula S, Kowalik I. Echocardiographic findings and 24-h electrocardiographic Holter monitoring in patients with nodular and non-nodular rheumatoid arthritis. Rheumatol Int 1999;18(5–6):163–9.
5. Rho YH, Chung CP, Oeser A, et al. Inflammatory mediators and premature coronary atherosclerosis in rheumatoid arthritis. Arthritis Rheum 2009;61(11): 1580–5.
6. Gullestad L, Aukrust P. Review of trials in chronic heart failure showing broad-spectrum anti-inflammatory approaches. Am J Cardiol 2005;95(11A):17C–23C [discussion: 38C–40C].
7. Chung CP, Giles JT, Petri M, et al. Prevalence of traditional modifiable cardiovascular risk factors in patients with rheumatoid arthritis: comparison with control subjects from the multi-ethnic study of atherosclerosis. Semin Arthritis Rheum 2012;41(4):535–44.
8. Meek IL, Picavet HS, Vonkeman HE, et al. Increased cardiovascular risk factors in different rheumatic diseases compared with the general population. Oxford (United Kingdom): Rheumatology; 2012.
9. Solomon DH, Curhan GC, Rimm EB, et al. Cardiovascular risk factors in women with and without rheumatoid arthritis. Arthritis Rheum 2004;50(11):3444–9.
10. del Rincon ID, Williams K, Stern MP, et al. High incidence of cardiovascular events in a rheumatoid arthritis cohort not explained by traditional cardiac risk factors. Arthritis Rheum 2001;44(12):2737–45.
11. Maradit-Kremers H, Nicola PJ, Crowson CS, et al. Cardiovascular death in rheumatoid arthritis: a population-based study. Arthritis Rheum 2005;52(3):722–32.
12. Guedes C, Bianchi-Fior P, Cormier B, et al. Cardiac manifestations of rheumatoid arthritis: a case-control transesophageal echocardiography study in 30 patients. Arthritis Rheum 2001;45(2):129–35.
13. Bonfiglio T, Atwater EC. Heart disease in patients with seropositive rheumatoid arthritis; a controlled autopsy study and review. Arch Intern Med 1969;124(6): 714–9.
14. Hansson GK. Inflammation, atherosclerosis, and coronary artery disease. N Engl J Med 2005;352(16):1685–95.
15. Costedoat-Chalumeau N, Hulot JS, Amoura Z, et al. Cardiomyopathy related to antimalarial therapy with illustrative case report. Cardiology 2007;107(2):73–80.
16. Bacani AK, Gabriel SE, Crowson CS, et al. Noncardiac vascular disease in rheumatoid arthritis: increase in venous thromboembolic events? Arthritis Rheum 2012;64(1):53–61.

17. Lindhardsen J, Ahlehoff O, Gislason GH, et al. Risk of atrial fibrillation and stroke in rheumatoid arthritis: danish nationwide cohort study. BMJ 2012;344:e1257.

18. Anker SD, Coats AJ. How to RECOVER from RENAISSANCE? The significance of the results of RECOVER, RENAISSANCE, RENEWAL and ATTACH. Int J Cardiol 2002;86(2–3):123–30.

19. Mann DL, McMurray JJ, Packer M, et al. Targeted anticytokine therapy in patients with chronic heart failure: results of the Randomized Etanercept Worldwide Evaluation (RENEWAL). Circulation 2004;109(13):1594–602.

20. Coletta AP, Clark AL, Banarjee P, et al. Clinical trials update: RENEWAL (RENAISSANCE and RECOVER) and ATTACH. Eur J Heart Fail 2002;4(4): 559–61.

21. Carmona L, Descalzo MA, Perez-Pampin E, et al. All-cause and cause-specific mortality in rheumatoid arthritis are not greater than expected when treated with tumour necrosis factor antagonists. Ann Rheum Dis 2007;66(7):880–5.

22. Wolfe F, Michaud K. Heart failure in rheumatoid arthritis: rates, predictors, and the effect of anti-tumor necrosis factor therapy. Am J Med 2004;116(5):305–11.

23. Singh JA, Furst DE, Bharat A, et al. 2012 update of the 2008 American College of Rheumatology recommendations for the use of disease-modifying antirheumatic drugs and biologic agents in the treatment of rheumatoid arthritis. Arthritis Care Res (Hoboken) 2012;64(5):625–39.

24. Greenberg JD, Kremer JM, Curtis JR, et al. Tumour necrosis factor antagonist use and associated risk reduction of cardiovascular events among patients with rheumatoid arthritis. Ann Rheum Dis 2011;70(4):576–82.

25. Dixon WG, Watson KD, Lunt M, et al. Reduction in the incidence of myocardial infarction in patients with rheumatoid arthritis who respond to anti-tumor necrosis factor alpha therapy: results from the British Society for Rheumatology Biologics Register. Arthritis Rheum 2007;56(9):2905–12.

26. Barnabe C, Martin BJ, Ghali WA. Systematic review and meta-analysis: anti-tumor necrosis factor alpha therapy and cardiovascular events in rheumatoid arthritis. Arthritis Care Res (Hoboken) 2011;63(4):522–9.

27. Raterman HG, Levels H, Voskuyl AE, et al. HDL protein composition alters from proatherogenic into less atherogenic and proinflammatory in rheumatoid arthritis patients responding to rituximab. Ann Rheum Dis 2012. [Epub ahead of print].

28. van Vollenhoven RF, Emery P, Bingham CO 3rd, et al. Longterm safety of patients receiving rituximab in rheumatoid arthritis clinical trials. J Rheumatol 2010;37(3):558–67.

29. Mathieu S. Assessment of Cardiovascular Markers after 24 weeks of Abatacept or Rituximab Therapy in patients with Rheumatoid Arthritis. Arthritis Rheum 2010;62(Suppl 3):388.

30. Maxwell L, Singh JA. Abatacept for rheumatoid arthritis. Cochrane Database Syst Rev 2009;(4):CD007277.

31. Hingorani AD, Casas JP. The interleukin-6 receptor as a target for prevention of coronary heart disease: a mendelian randomisation analysis. Lancet 2012; 379(9822):1214–24.

32. Emery P, Keystone E, Tony HP, et al. IL-6 receptor inhibition with tocilizumab improves treatment outcomes in patients with rheumatoid arthritis refractory to anti-tumour necrosis factor biologicals: results from a 24-week multicentre randomised placebo-controlled trial. Ann Rheum Dis 2008;67(11):1516–23.

33. Maini RN, Taylor PC, Szechinski J, et al. Double-blind randomized controlled clinical trial of the interleukin-6 receptor antagonist, tocilizumab, in European

patients with rheumatoid arthritis who had an incomplete response to methotrexate. Arthritis Rheum 2006;54(9):2817–29.

34. Smolen JS, Beaulieu A, Rubbert-Roth A, et al. Effect of interleukin-6 receptor inhibition with tocilizumab in patients with rheumatoid arthritis (OPTION study): a double-blind, placebo-controlled, randomised trial. Lancet 2008;371(9617): 987–97.

35. Nishimoto N, Miyasaka N, Yamamoto K, et al. Long-term safety and efficacy of tocilizumab, an anti-IL-6 receptor monoclonal antibody, in monotherapy, in patients with rheumatoid arthritis (the STREAM study): evidence of safety and efficacy in a 5-year extension study. Ann Rheum Dis 2009;68(10):1580–4.

36. Genovese MC, Sebba A. Long-Term Safety of Tocilizumab in Rheumatoid Arthritis Clinical Trials. Arthritis Rheum 2011;63(510):2217.

37. Schiff MH, DiVittorio G, Tesser J, et al. The safety of anakinra in high-risk patients with active rheumatoid arthritis: six-month observations of patients with comorbid conditions. Arthritis Rheum 2004;50(6):1752–60.

38. Bernatsky S, Hudson M, Suissa S. Anti-rheumatic drug use and risk of hospitalization for congestive heart failure in rheumatoid arthritis. Rheumatology (Oxford) 2005;44(5):677–80.

39. Suissa S, Bernatsky S, Hudson M. Antirheumatic drug use and the risk of acute myocardial infarction. Arthritis Rheum 2006;55(4):531–6.

40. Naranjo A, Sokka T, Descalzo MA, et al. Cardiovascular disease in patients with rheumatoid arthritis: results from the QUEST-RA study. Arthritis Res Ther 2008; 10(2):R30.

41. Choi HK, Hernan MA, Seeger JD, et al. Methotrexate and mortality in patients with rheumatoid arthritis: a prospective study. Lancet 2002;359(9313):1173–7.

42. Gong K, Zhang Z, Sun X, et al. The nonspecific anti-inflammatory therapy with methotrexate for patients with chronic heart failure. Am Heart J 2006;151(1): 62–8.

43. Micha R, Imamura F, Wyler von Ballmoos M, et al. Systematic review and meta-analysis of methotrexate use and risk of cardiovascular disease. Am J Cardiol 2011;108(9):1362–70.

44. Westlake SL, Colebatch AN, Baird J, et al. The effect of methotrexate on cardiovascular disease in patients with rheumatoid arthritis: a systematic literature review. Rheumatology (Oxford) 2010;49(2):295–307.

45. Estes ML, Ewing-Wilson D, Chou SM, et al. Chloroquine neuromyotoxicity. Clinical and pathologic perspective. Am J Med 1987;82(3):447–55.

46. Solomon DH, Avorn J, Katz JN, et al. Immunosuppressive medications and hospitalization for cardiovascular events in patients with rheumatoid arthritis. Arthritis Rheum 2006;54(12):3790–8.

47. Davis JM 3rd, Maradit Kremers H, Crowson CS, et al. Glucocorticoids and cardiovascular events in rheumatoid arthritis: a population-based cohort study. Arthritis Rheum 2007;56(3):820–30.

48. Mazzantini M, Talarico R, Doveri M, et al. Incident comorbidity among patients with rheumatoid arthritis treated or not with low-dose glucocorticoids: a retrospective study. J Rheumatol 2010;37(11):2232–6.

49. Souverein PC, Berard A, Van Staa TP, et al. Use of oral glucocorticoids and risk of cardiovascular and cerebrovascular disease in a population based case-control study. Heart 2004;90(8):859–65.

50. Antman EM, Bennett JS, Daugherty A, et al. Use of nonsteroidal antiinflammatory drugs: an update for clinicians: a scientific statement from the American Heart Association. Circulation 2007;115(12):1634–42.

51. Feenstra J, Heerdink ER, Grobbee DE, et al. Association of nonsteroidal anti-inflammatory drugs with first occurrence of heart failure and with relapsing heart failure: the Rotterdam Study. Arch Intern Med 2002;162(3):265–70.
52. Gislason GH, Rasmussen JN, Abildstrom SZ, et al. Increased mortality and cardiovascular morbidity associated with use of nonsteroidal anti-inflammatory drugs in chronic heart failure. Arch Intern Med 2009;169(2):141–9.
53. Aw TJ, Haas SJ, Liew D, et al. Meta-analysis of cyclooxygenase-2 inhibitors and their effects on blood pressure. Arch Intern Med 2005;165(5):490–6.
54. Chan CC, Reid CM, Aw TJ, et al. Do COX-2 inhibitors raise blood pressure more than nonselective NSAIDs and placebo? An updated meta-analysis. J Hypertens 2009;27(12):2332–41.
55. Trelle S, Reichenbach S, Wandel S, et al. Cardiovascular safety of non-steroidal anti-inflammatory drugs: network meta-analysis. BMJ 2011;342:c7086.
56. Pellicci PM, Ranawat CS, Tsairis P, et al. A prospective study of the progression of rheumatoid arthritis of the cervical spine. J Bone Joint Surg Am 1981;63(3):342–50.
57. Singleton JD, West SG, Reddy VV, et al. Cerebral vasculitis complicating rheumatoid arthritis. South Med J 1995;88(4):470–4.
58. Watson P, Fekete J, Deck J. Central nervous system vasculitis in rheumatoid arthritis. Can J Neurol Sci 1977;4(4):269–72.
59. Bathon JM, Moreland LW, DiBartolomeo AG. Inflammatory central nervous system involvement in rheumatoid arthritis. Semin Arthritis Rheum 1989;18(4):258–66.
60. Bernatsky S, Renoux C, Suissa S. Demyelinating events in rheumatoid arthritis after drug exposures. Ann Rheum Dis 2010;69(9):1691–3.
61. Midgard R, Gronning M, Riise T, et al. Multiple sclerosis and chronic inflammatory diseases. A case-control study. Acta Neurol Scand 1996;93(5):322–8.
62. Toussirot E, Pertuiset E, Martin A, et al. Association of rheumatoid arthritis with multiple sclerosis: report of 14 cases and discussion of its significance. J Rheumatol 2006;33(5):1027–8.
63. Mohan N, Edwards ET, Cupps TR, et al. Demyelination occurring during anti-tumor necrosis factor alpha therapy for inflammatory arthritides. Arthritis Rheum 2001;44(12):2862–9.
64. Simsek I, Erdem H, Pay S, et al. Optic neuritis occurring with anti-tumour necrosis factor alpha therapy. Ann Rheum Dis 2007;66(9):1255–8.
65. Gabriel SE, Crowson CS, O'Fallon WM. Comorbidity in arthritis. J Rheumatol 1999;26(11):2475–9.
66. Olson AL, Swigris JJ, Sprunger DB, et al. Rheumatoid arthritis-interstitial lung disease-associated mortality. Am J Respir Crit Care Med 2011;183(3):372–8.
67. Antohe JL, Bili A, Sartorius JA, et al. Diabetes mellitus risk in rheumatoid arthritis: reduced incidence with anti-tumor necrosis factor alpha therapy. Arthritis Care Res (Hoboken) 2012;64(2):215–21.
68. Mork NL, Robertson RP. Effects of nonsteroidal antiinflammatory drugs in conventional dosage on glucose homeostasis in patients with diabetes. West J Med 1983;139(1):46–9.
69. Dessein PH, Joffe BI, Stanwix AE, et al. Glucocorticoids and insulin sensitivity in rheumatoid arthritis. J Rheumatol 2004;31(5):867–74.
70. Pincus T, Castrejon I, Sokka T. Long-term prednisone in doses of less than 5 mg/day for treatment of rheumatoid arthritis: personal experience over 25 years. Clin Exp Rheumatol 2011;29(5 Suppl 68):S130–8.
71. Panthakalam S, Bhatnagar D, Klimiuk P. The prevalence and management of hyperglycaemia in patients with rheumatoid arthritis on corticosteroid therapy. Scott Med J 2004;49(4):139–41.

72. Penn SK, Kao AH, Schott LL, et al. Hydroxychloroquine and glycemia in women with rheumatoid arthritis and systemic lupus erythematosus. J Rheumatol 2010; 37(6):1136–42.
73. Rekedal LR, Massarotti E, Garg R, et al. Changes in glycosylated hemoglobin after initiation of hydroxychloroquine or methotrexate treatment in diabetes patients with rheumatic diseases. Arthritis Rheum 2010;62(12):3569–73.
74. Haas RM, Li P, Chu JW. Glucose-lowering effects of sulfasalazine in type 2 diabetes. Diabetes Care 2005;28(9):2238–9.
75. Araujo EP, De Souza CT, Ueno M, et al. Infliximab restores glucose homeostasis in an animal model of diet-induced obesity and diabetes. Endocrinology 2007; 148(12):5991–7.
76. Gupta-Ganguli M, Cox K, Means B, et al. Does therapy with anti-TNF-alpha improve glucose tolerance and control in patients with type 2 diabetes? Diabetes Care 2011;34(7):e121.
77. Komano Y, Tanaka M, Nanki T, et al. Incidence and risk factors for serious infection in patients with rheumatoid arthritis treated with tumor necrosis factor inhibitors: a report from the Registry of Japanese Rheumatoid Arthritis Patients for Longterm Safety. J Rheumatol 2011;38(7):1258–64.
78. Larsen CM, Faulenbach M, Vaag A, et al. Interleukin-1-receptor antagonist in type 2 diabetes mellitus. N Engl J Med 2007;356(15):1517–26.
79. Schultz O, Oberhauser F, Saech J, et al. Effects of inhibition of interleukin-6 signalling on insulin sensitivity and lipoprotein (a) levels in human subjects with rheumatoid diseases. PLoS One 2010;5(12):e14328.
80. Cortet B, Perez T, Roux N, et al. Pulmonary function tests and high resolution computed tomography of the lungs in patients with rheumatoid arthritis. Ann Rheum Dis 1997;56(10):596–600.
81. Dawson JK, Fewins HE, Desmond J, et al. Fibrosing alveolitis in patients with rheumatoid arthritis as assessed by high resolution computed tomography, chest radiography, and pulmonary function tests. Thorax 2001;56(8):622–7.
82. Fewins HE, McGowan I, Whitehouse GH, et al. High definition computed tomography in rheumatoid arthritis associated pulmonary disease. Br J Rheumatol 1991;30(3):214–6.
83. Gabbay E, Tarala R, Will R, et al. Interstitial lung disease in recent onset rheumatoid arthritis. Am J Respir Crit Care Med 1997;156(2 Pt 1):528–35.
84. McDonagh J, Greaves M, Wright AR, et al. High resolution computed tomography of the lungs in patients with rheumatoid arthritis and interstitial lung disease. Br J Rheumatol 1994;33(2):118–22.
85. Lee HK, Kim DS, Yoo B, et al. Histopathologic pattern and clinical features of rheumatoid arthritis-associated interstitial lung disease. Chest 2005;127(6): 2019–27.
86. Bongartz T, Nannini C, Medina-Velasquez YF, et al. Incidence and mortality of interstitial lung disease in rheumatoid arthritis: a population-based study. Arthritis Rheum 2010;62(6):1583–91.
87. Raghu G, Depaso WJ, Cain K, et al. Azathioprine combined with prednisone in the treatment of idiopathic pulmonary fibrosis: a prospective double-blind, randomized, placebo-controlled clinical trial. Am Rev Respir Dis 1991;144(2):291–6.
88. Saketkoo LA, Espinoza LR. Rheumatoid arthritis interstitial lung disease: mycophenolate mofetil as an antifibrotic and disease-modifying antirheumatic drug. Arch Intern Med 2008;168(15):1718–9.
89. Malik S, Saravanan V, Kelly C. Interstitial lung disease in rheumatoid arthritis: an update on diagnosis and management. Int J Clin Rheumatol 2012;7(3):297–308.

90. Wolfe F, Mitchell DM, Sibley JT, et al. The mortality of rheumatoid arthritis. Arthritis Rheum 1994;37(4):481–94.
91. Hargreaves MR, Mowat AG, Benson MK. Acute pneumonitis associated with low dose methotrexate treatment for rheumatoid arthritis: report of five cases and review of published reports. Thorax 1992;47(8):628–33.
92. Bell MJ, Geddie WR, Gordon DA, et al. Pre-existing lung disease in patients with rheumatoid arthritis may predispose to methotrexate lung. Arthritis Rheum 1987; 29:S75.
93. St Clair EW, Rice JR, Snyderman R. Pneumonitis complicating low-dose methotrexate therapy in rheumatoid arthritis. Arch Intern Med 1985;145(11):2035–8.
94. Newman ED, Harrington TM. Fatal methotrexate pneumonitis in rheumatoid arthritis. Arthritis Rheum 1988;31(12):1585–6.
95. Golden MR, Katz RS, Balk RA, et al. The relationship of preexisting lung disease to the development of methotrexate pneumonitis in patients with rheumatoid arthritis. J Rheumatol 1995;22(6):1043–7.
96. Ridley MG, Wolfe CS, Mathews JA. Life threatening acute pneumonitis during low dose methotrexate treatment for rheumatoid arthritis: a case report and review of the literature. Ann Rheum Dis 1988;47(9):784–8.
97. Searles G, McKendry RJ. Methotrexate pneumonitis in rheumatoid arthritis: potential risk factors. Four case reports and a review of the literature. J Rheumatol 1987;14(6):1164–71.
98. Ohosone Y, Okano Y, Kameda H, et al. Clinical characteristics of patients with rheumatoid arthritis and methotrexate induced pneumonitis. J Rheumatol 1997;24(12):2299–303.
99. Methotrexate in rheumatoid arthritis. Health and Public Policy Committee, American College of Physicians. Ann Intern Med 1987;107(3):418–9.
100. Mandel MA. The synergistic effect of salicylates on methotrexate toxicity. Plast Reconstr Surg 1976;57(6):733–7.
101. Carson CW, Cannon GW, Egger MJ, et al. Pulmonary disease during the treatment of rheumatoid arthritis with low dose pulse methotrexate. Semin Arthritis Rheum 1987;16(3):186–95.
102. Cook NJ, Carroll GJ. Successful reintroduction of methotrexate after pneumonitis in two patients with rheumatoid arthritis. Ann Rheum Dis 1992;51(2): 272–4.
103. Kamata Y, Nara H, Kamimura T, et al. Rheumatoid arthritis complicated with acute interstitial pneumonia induced by leflunomide as an adverse reaction. Intern Med 2004;43(12):1201–4.
104. Parry SD, Barbatzas C, Peel ET, et al. Sulphasalazine and lung toxicity. Eur Respir J 2002;19(4):756–64.
105. Perez-Alvarez R, Perez-de-Lis M, Diaz-Lagares C, et al. Interstitial lung disease induced or exacerbated by TNF-targeted therapies: analysis of 122 cases. Semin Arthritis Rheum 2011;41(2):256–64.
106. Wynn TA. Fibrotic disease and the T(H)1/T(H)2 paradigm. Nat Rev Immunol 2004;4(8):583–94.
107. Dixon WG, Hyrich KL, Watson KD, et al. Influence of anti-TNF therapy on mortality in patients with rheumatoid arthritis-associated interstitial lung disease: results from the British Society for Rheumatology Biologics Register. Ann Rheum Dis 2010;69(6):1086–91.
108. Kawashiri SY, Kawakami A, Sakamoto N, et al. A fatal case of acute exacerbation of interstitial lung disease in a patient with rheumatoid arthritis during treatment with tocilizumab. Rheumatol Int 2010. [Epub ahead of print].

109. Storage SS, Agrawal H, Furst DE. Description of the efficacy and safety of three new biologics in the treatment of rheumatoid arthritis. Korean J Intern Med 2010; 25(1):1–17.

110. Kremer JM, Dougados M, Emery P, et al. Treatment of rheumatoid arthritis with the selective costimulation modulator abatacept: twelve-month results of a phase iib, double-blind, randomized, placebo-controlled trial. Arthritis Rheum 2005;52(8):2263–71.

111. Weinblatt M, Combe B, Covucci A, et al. Safety of the selective costimulation modulator abatacept in rheumatoid arthritis patients receiving background biologic and nonbiologic disease-modifying antirheumatic drugs: a one-year randomized, placebo-controlled study. Arthritis Rheum 2006;54(9):2807–16.

112. Liote H, Liote F, Seroussi B, et al. Rituximab-induced lung disease: a systematic literature review. Eur Respir J 2010;35(3):681–7.

113. Wagner SA, Mehta AC, Laber DA. Rituximab-induced interstitial lung disease. Am J Hematol 2007;82(10):916–9.

114. Emery P, Fleischmann R, Filipowicz-Sosnowska A, et al. The efficacy and safety of rituximab in patients with active rheumatoid arthritis despite methotrexate treatment: results of a phase IIB randomized, double-blind, placebo-controlled, dose-ranging trial. Arthritis Rheum 2006;54(5):1390–400.

115. Matteson EL, Dellaripa, PF, Ryu, JH, et al. Open-label, pilot study of the safety and clinical effects of rituximab in patients with rheumatoid arthritis-associated interstitial pneumonia. Open J Rheumatol Autoimmunity, in press.

116. Boers M, Dijkmans BA, Breedveld FC, et al. Errors in the prediction of creatinine clearance in patients with rheumatoid arthritis. Br J Rheumatol 1988;27(3): 233–5.

117. Boers M. Renal disorders in rheumatoid arthritis. Semin Arthritis Rheum 1990; 20(1):57–68.

118. Scott DG, Bacon PA. Intravenous cyclophosphamide plus methylprednisolone in treatment of systemic rheumatoid vasculitis. Am J Med 1984;76(3):377–84.

119. Scott DG, Bacon PA, Elliott PJ, et al. Systemic vasculitis in a district general hospital 1972-1980: clinical and laboratory features, classification and prognosis of 80 cases. Q J Med 1982;51(203):292–311.

120. Laakso M, Mutru O, Isomaki H, et al. Mortality from amyloidosis and renal diseases in patients with rheumatoid arthritis. Ann Rheum Dis 1986;45(8):663–7.

121. Rasker JJ, Cosh JA. Cause and age at death in a prospective study of 100 patients with rheumatoid arthritis. Ann Rheum Dis 1981;40(2):115–20.

122. Sihvonen S, Korpela M, Mustonen J, et al. Renal disease as a predictor of increased mortality among patients with rheumatoid arthritis. Nephron Clin Pract 2004;96(4):c107–14.

123. Koseki Y, Terai C, Moriguchi M, et al. A prospective study of renal disease in patients with early rheumatoid arthritis. Ann Rheum Dis 2001;60(4):327–31.

124. Karie S, Gandjbakhch F, Janus N, et al. Kidney disease in RA patients: prevalence and implication on RA-related drugs management: the MATRIX study. Rheumatology (Oxford) 2008;47(3):350–4.

125. Helin HJ, Korpela MM, Mustonen JT, et al. Renal biopsy findings and clinicopathologic correlations in rheumatoid arthritis. Arthritis Rheum 1995;38(2):242–7.

126. Nakano M, Ueno M, Nishi S, et al. Analysis of renal pathology and drug history in 158 Japanese patients with rheumatoid arthritis. Clin Nephrol 1998;50(3):154–60.

127. Orjavik O, Brodwall EK, Oystese B, et al. A renal biopsy study with light and immunofluorescent microscopy in rheumatoid arthritis. Acta Med Scand Suppl 1981;645:9–14.

128. Salomon MI, Gallo G, Poon TP, et al. The kidney in rheumatoid arthritis. A study based on renal biopsies. Nephron 1974;12(4):297–310.
129. Brun C, Olsen TS, Raaschou F, et al. Renal biopsy in rheumatoid arthritis. Nephron 1965;2(2):65–81.
130. Horl W. Nonsteroidal anti-inflammatory drugs and the kidney. Pharmaceuticals 2010;3(7):2291–321.
131. Whelton A. Nephrotoxicity of nonsteroidal anti-inflammatory drugs: physiologic foundations and clinical implications. Am J Med 1999;106(5B):13S–24S.
132. Schiff MH, Whelton A. Renal toxicity associated with disease-modifying anti-rheumatic drugs used for the treatment of rheumatoid arthritis. Semin Arthritis Rheum 2000;30(3):196–208.
133. Mason J. The effect of cyclosporin on renal function. J Autoimmun 1992;5(Suppl A): 349–54.
134. Breedveld FC, Markusse HM, MacFarlane JD. Subcutaneous fat biopsy in the diagnosis of amyloidosis secondary to chronic arthritis. Clin Exp Rheumatol 1989;7(4):407–10.
135. Cush JJ, Tugwell P, Weinblatt M, et al. US consensus guidelines for the use of cyclosporin A in rheumatoid arthritis. J Rheumatol 1999;26(5):1176–86.
136. Kremer JM, Petrillo GF, Hamilton RA. Pharmacokinetics and renal function in patients with rheumatoid arthritis receiving a standard dose of oral weekly methotrexate: association with significant decreases in creatinine clearance and renal clearance of the drug after 6 months of therapy. J Rheumatol 1995; 22(1):38–40.
137. Seideman P, Muller-Suur R, Ekman E. Renal effects of low dose methotrexate in rheumatoid arthritis. J Rheumatol 1993;20(7):1126–8.
138. The effect of age and renal function on the efficacy and toxicity of methotrexate in rheumatoid arthritis. Rheumatoid Arthritis Clinical Trial Archive Group. J Rheumatol 1995;22(2):218–23.
139. Landewe RB, Vergouwen MS, Goeei The SG, et al. Antimalarial drug induced decrease in creatinine clearance. J Rheumatol 1995;22(1):34–7.
140. Mackenzie AH. Dose refinements in long-term therapy of rheumatoid arthritis with antimalarials. Am J Med 1983;75(1A):40–5.
141. Sulfasalazine in early rheumatoid arthritis. The Australian Multicentre Clinical Trial Group. J Rheumatol 1992;19(11):1672–7.
142. Smolen JS, Kalden JR, Scott DL, et al. Efficacy and safety of leflunomide compared with placebo and sulphasalazine in active rheumatoid arthritis: a double-blind, randomised, multicentre trial. European Leflunomide Study Group. Lancet 1999;353(9149):259–66.
143. Strand V, Cohen S, Schiff M, et al. Treatment of active rheumatoid arthritis with leflunomide compared with placebo and methotrexate. Leflunomide Rheumatoid Arthritis Investigators Group. Arch Intern Med 1999;159(21):2542–50.
144. Singh G, Fries JF, Spitz P, et al. Toxic effects of azathioprine in rheumatoid arthritis. A national post-marketing perspective. Arthritis Rheum 1989;32(7): 837–43.
145. Whisnant JK, Pelkey J. Rheumatoid arthritis: treatment with azathioprine (IMURAN (R)). Clinical side-effects and laboratory abnormalities. Ann Rheum Dis 1982;41(Suppl 1):44–7.
146. Beaman JM, Hackett LP, Luxton G, et al. Effect of hemodialysis on leflunomide plasma concentrations. Ann Pharmacother 2002;36(1):75–7.
147. Meibohm B, Zhou H. Characterizing the impact of renal impairment on the clinical pharmacology of biologics. J Clin Pharmacol 2012;52(Suppl 1):54S–62S.

Comparative Safety of Therapies in Systemic Lupus Erythematosus

Joseph Mosak, MD[a],*, Richard Furie, MD[a,b]

KEYWORDS

- Systemic lupus erythematosus • Adverse effects • Antimalarials • Azathioprine
- Cyclophosphamide • Mycophenolate mofetil • Rituximab • Belimumab

KEY POINTS

- A wide variety of medications are used to treat systemic lupus erythematosus, depending on organ involvement and severity.
- Some of these drugs, especially immunosuppressive and cytotoxic agents, often lead to significant toxicity.
- Physicians must familiarize themselves with the adverse effects of each of these drugs and discuss them with patients to facilitate educated decision making.

Systemic lupus erythematosus (SLE) is the prototypic autoimmune disease resulting from a dysregulation of immune function. Diverse clinical manifestations may be seen, affecting virtually all organ systems.[1] For this reason, a wide variety of medications are used for treatment, depending on organ involvement and severity. Although some of these treatments are usually safe and well tolerated, others, especially immunosuppressive and cytotoxic agents, often lead to significant toxicity.

ANTIMALARIALS

Several antimalarial medications have been used to treat SLE for more than 100 years. Hydroxychloroquine (Plaquenil) is currently the most commonly used, although chloroquine (Aralen) and quinacrine (Atabrine, Mepacrine) also remain in use. Several recent studies have highlighted the many benefits of antimalarials in patients with SLE, including

- An improvement in lipid profiles[2]
- Reduction of SLE activity[3]

Disclosure: Dr Furie has served as a paid consultant to: 1) Genentech, Roche, and Biogenidec; 2) Human Genome Sciences, GlaxoSmithKline.
Funding sources: None.
Conflicts of interest: None.
[a] Division of Rheumatology and Allergy-Clinical Immunology, North Shore–Long Island Jewish Health System, 2800 Marcus Avenue, Suite 200, Lake Success, NY 11042, USA; [b] Hofstra North Shore–Long Island Jewish School of Medicine, Hofstra University, Hempstead, NY, USA
* Corresponding author.
E-mail address: jmosak@nshs.edu

- Prevention of thrombotic events[3]
- Improved survival[4,5]

Although antimalarials are generally well tolerated and possess good safety profiles, they are associated with adverse events (AEs), although these are infrequent and generally mild. The most common AEs are gastrointestinal and cutaneous, whereas the most serious AE, although rare, is retinopathy. In one study comparing the toxicities associated with hydroxychloroquine and chloroquine, 28% of patients receiving chloroquine experienced AEs compared with 15% of those receiving hydroxychloroquine (P<.00001).[6]

Retinopathy

The risk of retinopathy (**Fig. 1**) from hydroxychloroquine is low, especially compared with chloroquine. In a study performed in Thailand, 37 of 139 patients (27%) receiving chloroquine experienced retinopathy.[7] In contrast, in a large series of 1207 patients taking hydroxychloroquine for rheumatic diseases, only 1 case of definite retinal toxicity was identified.[8] In a more recent study, definite or probable retinal toxicity occurred in 0.65% of 3995 patients taking hydroxychloroquine. Although the toxicity rate remained low with longer durations, an increase in toxicity was seen after approximately 6 years of use, or with a cumulative dose of 800 g.[9] For this reason, the American Academy of Ophthalmology recommends that all patients starting on hydroxychloroquine or chloroquine have a baseline examination within the first year of starting the drug. Annual screening should then be performed after 5 years of use in all patients, and from initiation of therapy for patients with maculopathy or unusual risk factors.[10] Recommended screening procedures include careful ocular examination, automated visual field testing, and, when available, testing with one or more objective tests of anatomic or functional damage.

Cutaneous

Cutaneous side effects are common in patients taking antimalarials. Cutaneous pigmentary changes have been found in up to 25% of patients taking these medications for more than 3 months.[11] Any of the antimalarials may produce localized blue-black pigmentation, which predominantly affects the pretibial areas, face, gums, hard palate, and subungual regions, although it has most commonly been seen with chloroquine (**Figs. 2** and **3**).[12] This effect was seen in 25 of 300 patients receiving

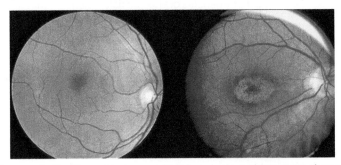

Fig. 1. Left: an early "bull's-eye" lesion resulted from hydroxychloroquine therapy. Stippled annular hyperpigmentation of the macula is seen. Right: a late lesion shows a central area of hyperpigmentation and an intermediate zone of hypopigmentation encircled by a pigmented rim, creating the characteristic bull's-eye effect. (© 2012 American College of Rheumatology. Used with permission.)

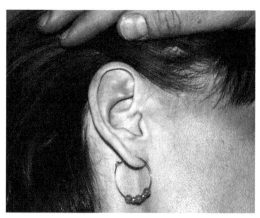

Fig. 2. Blue-gray hyperpigmentation of the ear. (© 2012 American College of Rheumatology. Used with permission.)

antimalarials for collagen diseases. Early lesions resembled ecchymoses, but with continued therapy, the areas coalesced and became darker. The duration of therapy varied from 4 to 70 months, and the pigmentation decreased several months after cessation of therapy. African Americans seemed to have a lower incidence of pigmentary changes.[13]

In addition, quinacrine may cause a generalized lemon-yellow discoloration of the skin, with varying degrees of severity. This pigmentation fades within 4 months of discontinuation.

Gastrointestinal

Gastrointestinal side effects are the most common reason for discontinuing antimalarials. In a recent study, 28% of 869 patients started on antimalarials discontinued use because of AEs. Of these AEs, 44.5% were ophthalmologic. Of the nonophthalmologic AEs leading to discontinuation, 43.5% were gastrointestinal. Median treatment survival was 8.38 years. Sixty-eight percent of the discontinuations occurred during the first year of treatment. No significant difference in discontinuation rates was found between patients on hydroxychloroquine and those on chloroquine.[14]

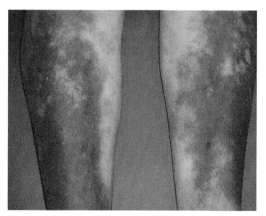

Fig. 3. Blue-gray skin pigmentation as a result of chronic hydroxychloroquine therapy. (© 2012 American College of Rheumatology. Used with permission.)

Nausea is most common, whereas vomiting and diarrhea also occasionally occur. Hepatotoxicity is rare, although the literature contains case reports of 3 patients who developed acute liver failure soon after starting hydroxychloroquine.[15,16] In one of these cases, the patient improved quickly after discontinuation of hydroxychloroquine and was later started on chloroquine with no further liver toxicity.

Other AEs

Other less common AEs reported in patients taking antimalarials include:

- Central nervous system (CNS) involvement: headaches are the most common CNS AE, followed by lightheadedness. One case series reports 3 patients who experienced neuropsychiatric disturbances, ranging from restlessness, insomnia, and hyperirritability to frank psychosis and seizures, while taking quinacrine.[17]
- Cardiotoxicity: several case reports have described antimalarials causing cardiotoxicity, including cardiomyopathy or conduction abnormalities; these reports have been more common with chloroquine than hydroxychloroquine.[18,19]
- Myopathy (**Fig. 4**).

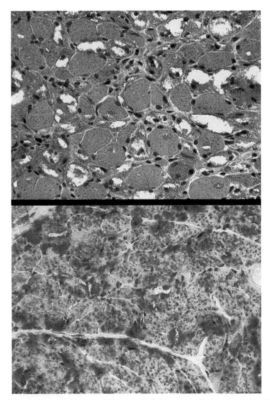

Fig. 4. Top: typical vacuolar degeneration involving multiple muscle fibers is present in chloroquine-induced myopathy. Marked fiber size variation is seen (hematoxylin-eosin, medium power). Bottom: increased acid phosphatase activity (*red*) is seen within the vacuoles because of their autophagic nature (acid phosphatase, medium power). (© 2012 American College of Rheumatology. Used with permission.)

Pregnancy

Antimalarials are considered safe during pregnancy. In a systematic review of the literature, 10 studies were found on the effects of antimalarials on children born to mothers with lupus. Of 311 pregnant patients, no significant toxicity was reported, and congenital malformations were no more frequent than in unexposed children.[3]

AZATHIOPRINE (IMURAN, AZASAN)

At the doses typically used for patients with SLE, the most common AEs with azathioprine are infection, bone marrow suppression, and gastrointestinal side effects, although other less common AEs also must be kept in mind.

Bone Marrow Suppression

Leukopenia can be seen in up to 29% of patients receiving azathioprine, whereas thrombocytopenia occurs less frequently. This AE can normally be reversed with a dose reduction.[20] The enzyme thiopurine methyltransferase (TPMT) is responsible for the conversion of the active metabolites of azathioprine, 6-mercaptopurine (6-MP) and thioinosine monophosphate, to inactive metabolites (**Fig. 5**). In patients with subnormal TPMT activity, concentrations of 6-thioguanine nucleotides (6-TGNs) increase. Their levels correlate inversely with 6-TGN levels in erythrocytes (low TPMT results in high 6-TGN and greater marrow cytotoxicity, whereas high TPMT results in low 6-TGN and less marrow cytotoxicity). In the approximately 0.3% of the population who are deficient in this enzyme, azathioprine can result in serious myelosuppression; therefore, the drug should be avoided. For the 10% of the population that is heterozygous, a 50% dose reduction should occur. TPMT screening can be accomplished via 2 different methods: genotyping or phenotyping. Although each has its disadvantages, phenotyping is more commonly used. Some experts recommend a combination of phenotyping with supportive genotyping.[21]

Caution must also be used in patients undergoing treatment with the xanthine oxidase inhibitors allopurinol and, more recently, febuxostat. Xanthine oxidase converts 6-MP to thiouric acid. Inhibition of xanthine oxidase, therefore, potentiates the action of 6-MP and can lead to serious myelosuppression.[22] Allopurinol and febuxostat should therefore be avoided in patients being treated with azathioprine.

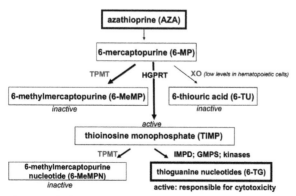

Fig. 5. Azathioprine metabolism. GMPS, guanosine monophosphate synthetase; HGPRT, hypoxanthine-guanine-phosphoribosyl-transferase; IMPD, inosine monophosphate dehydrogenase; TPMT, thiopurine S-methyltransferase; XO, xanthine oxidase.

In patients with severe gout who cannot be taken off xanthine oxidase inhibitors, the azathioprine dose should be reduced by 50% and blood counts should be carefully monitored.

Gastrointestinal

The most common gastrointestinal AEs in patients receiving azathioprine are nausea, anorexia, and vomiting, usually occurring within the first few weeks of treatment. Although these symptoms do not seem to be dose-related, they generally respond rapidly to cessation of treatment.[20] One of the authors (RF) has successfully used 6-MP to treat patients who developed significant diarrhea and vomiting from azathioprine; recurrent symptoms were averted with this approach. Mild elevation of liver enzymes may sometimes occur, and liver function tests should therefore be monitored regularly.

Infections

Although infections occur frequently in patients receiving azathioprine, serious infections are less common. In the recently completed maintenance phase of the Aspreva Lupus Management Study (ALMS) trial, 78.4% of patients receiving azathioprine experienced infections compared with 79.1% in the mycophenolate mofetil (MMF) arm, whereas the rate of serious infections was 11.7% with azathioprine compared with 9.6% with MMF.[23] Herpes zoster is a common viral infection in patients receiving azathioprine.[20] Reactivation of chronic viral hepatitis has been described, and caution must therefore be used in this population.[24]

Pregnancy

Studies of pregnant patients receiving azathioprine have not shown a significant increase in pregnancy complications or congenital malformations. Several reports exist of intrauterine growth restriction in patients on a combination of corticosteroids and azathioprine. If an immunosuppressive is required during pregnancy, it is generally accepted that azathioprine can be prescribed at a daily dose not exceeding 2 mg/kg/d.[25]

CYCLOPHOSPHAMIDE (CYTOXAN)

Although it remains one of the most effective medications for the treatment of SLE, cyclophosphamide also can lead to a variety of AEs. The most serious include malignancy and infertility. Others include infection, hemorrhagic cystitis, and bone marrow suppression.

Malignancy

Patients treated with cyclophosphamide are at an increased risk for developing malignancies, especially bladder cancer, skin cancer, and hematologic malignancies. In one long-term study of patients with rheumatoid arthritis (RA), 31% treated with cyclophosphamide developed malignancies, compared with 21% in the control group ($P<.05$). Of a total of 51 malignancies identified in the cyclophosphamide group, 19 were skin cancer (vs 6 in the control group), 9 were bladder cancer (vs 0 in the control group), and 5 were myeloproliferative (vs 1 in the control group).[26] Another study showed that patients with SLE treated with cyclophosphamide had adjusted hazard ratios of 1.16 for all malignancies and 2.09 for hematologic malignancies, although these increased risks did not reach statistical significance.[27] Finally, in a cohort of patients with RA, those treated with cyclophosphamide had an adjusted hazard ratio of 1.84 for developing hematologic malignancies compared with controls, a result that reached statistical significance in this study.[28]

Bone Marrow Suppression

Although cytopenias occur frequently in patients receiving cyclophosphamide, severe leukopenia is much less common. In a study comparing intravenous and oral cyclophosphamide for the treatment of lupus nephritis, 5% and 7% of patients, respectively, developed severe leukopenia (white blood cell count <2000/μL).[29] Concomitant administration of corticosteroids helps spare the bone marrow–suppressive effects of cyclophosphamide; however, physicians should exercise an extra degree of laboratory surveillance when the steroids are tapered to low doses. A reduction in the cyclophosphamide dose might be required.

Infections

Infections are common in patients treated with cyclophosphamide. In the induction phase of the ALMS trial, 61.7% of patients in the cyclophosphamide arm developed infections.[30] Bacterial infections are the most common, followed by opportunistic infections and herpes zoster. In an earlier study of infection rates in patients on cyclophosphamide, opportunistic infections and herpes zoster were more common in patients with SLE with multiple organ disease than in those with single organ disease. The route of administration of cyclophosphamide had no effect on infection rates. A white blood count nadir of less than 3000 cells/μL at any point during the course of treatment was found to be a significant risk factor for infection.[31]

Gonadal Toxicity

Because SLE primarily affects women in their childbearing years, the complication about which patients are often most concerned is premature ovarian failure (POF). This effect of cyclophosphamide on reproductive capacity has been reported in multiple studies.[32,33] The 10-year follow-up data from the Euro-Lupus Nephritis Trial showed no difference in pregnancy rates between the National Institutes of Health (NIH; "high-dose") and Euro-Lupus ("low-dose") protocols (9 of 46 patients in the NIH arm experienced successful pregnancies compared with 10 of 44 in the Euro-Lupus arm).[34] The risk of POF has been shown to be related to age (greatest risk, >30 years of age) and duration of treatment (greatest risk, >15 doses of pulse cyclophosphamide).[35] Similarly, in patients with SLE treated with oral cyclophosphamide, the risk of amenorrhea was found to be associated with older age at the initiation of treatment and with the cumulative dose.[36] Administration of gonadotropin-releasing hormone (GnRH) analogs (depot injections of 3.75 mg/mo administered 10 days before each cyclophosphamide dose) to induce gonadal quiescence has been shown to significantly reduce the risk of POF.[37,38] After 4 weeks of therapy, patients without contraindications were given an estradiol patch (estradiol transdermal system, 0.05 or 0.1 mg) to maintain estrogen at slightly less than early follicular phase levels and to reduce symptoms of hormonal withdrawal.

Although far fewer studies have been conducted on men receiving cyclophosphamide, men also seem to experience a high risk of infertility. In one study of 30 men treated with cyclophosphamide, 4 developed azoospermia and 9 oligospermia after a mean follow-up of 12.8 years.[39] Less is known about prevention of gonadal toxicity in men, because no large studies have been performed. No benefit from the administration of GnRH analogs was shown.[23,40] Several small studies examining the effects of the concomitant administration of testosterone suggested that fertility may be preserved with this treatment approach.[41,42]

Bladder Toxicity

Acrolein, a toxic metabolite of cyclophosphamide, is injurious to the bladder epithelium and is responsible for both bladder cancer and hemorrhagic cystitis. The risk for both of these is much higher in patients treated with oral compared with intravenous cyclophosphamide. Although 2-mercaptoethane sulfonate sodium (mesna) is commonly used to prevent cystitis and bladder cancer, evidence of its effectiveness is largely based on its use with the alkylating agent ifosfamide in patients with cancer. The value of mesna in patients with SLE receiving cyclophosphamide is unclear.[43]

Pregnancy

Cyclophosphamide is contraindicated during pregnancy.

MYCOPHENOLATE MOFETIL (CELLCEPT)

The most common AEs in patients receiving MMF are gastrointestinal, infectious, and bone marrow suppression. In one study, 67% of patients with SLE receiving MMF experienced AEs, although most were mild, and only 17% of study subjects discontinued treatment as a result.[44] Similarly, in the ALMS trial, 96% of patients receiving MMF reported AEs, although only 13% withdrew from the study as a result.[30]

Gastrointestinal

Gastrointestinal toxicities, which are generally dose-related, include nausea, vomiting, diarrhea, and, less commonly, abdominal pain or cramping.[44] In some patients, these may improve by distributing the daily dose in smaller, more frequent doses (3 times per day), whereas others may require a reduction in the total daily dose. Some patients may benefit from being converted to treatment with enteric-coated mycophenolate sodium (EC-MPS; Myfortic). In a study of renal transplant recipients, only 10% of patients who had been converted to EC-MPS required a dose reduction during 6 months of observation.[45]

Infections

Infections are fairly common, although usually minor. In the study mentioned earlier, 24 of 54 (44%) patients with SLE receiving MMF experienced a total of 37 infectious AEs.[44] In the maintenance phase of the ALMS trial, 79.1% of patients experienced infections, although the rate of serious infections was just 9.6%.[46]

Bone Marrow Suppression

MMF has been associated with cytopenias, especially leukopenia, and therefore requires monitoring of blood counts.

Pregnancy

MMF is contraindicated during pregnancy.

RITUXIMAB (RITUXAN)

In the Explorer trial, the most common AE in patients receiving rituximab was an infusion reaction (43.8% of patients), followed by infections (9.5%), musculoskeletal and connective tissue disorders (5.3%), gastrointestinal disorders (4.7%), neutropenia (3.6%), and cardiac disorders (3.0%). However, all of these AEs, except infusion reactions and neutropenia, were actually more frequent in the placebo group than the rituximab group.[47]

Similarly, in the recently published Lupus Nephritis Assessment With Rituximab trial, AEs occurred with similar frequency in the rituximab and placebo arms, whereas serious AEs were more frequent in the placebo group. Neutropenia, leukopenia, hypotension, and infusion reactions related to study drug (16.4%) were more frequent in the rituximab group.[48]

Progressive Multifocal Leukoencephalopathy

There have been multiple reports, including a case series of 57 patients, of patients on rituximab who developed progressive multifocal leukoencephalopathy (PML). Most of these patients were being treated for lymphoproliferative disorders, although 2 had SLE. The pathophysiology of rituximab-associated PML remains unclear.[49]

Hypogammaglobulinemia

Several studies have shown that patients treated with repeated courses of rituximab are at an increased risk of developing hypogammaglobulinemia, although the rate of infection in these patients was comparable to that in those whose immunoglobulin levels remained normal.[50,51]

Pregnancy

Rituximab is not recommended during pregnancy.

BELIMUMAB (BENLYSTA)

Belimumab was approved by the U.S. Food and Drug Administration in 2011 for patients with SLE based on favorable results from 2 large phase III studies, BLISS-52 and BLISS-76. Belimumab was generally well tolerated in both of these studies, in which the total numbers of adverse events in the belimumab and placebo groups were nearly identical. The overall rates of infection and rates of serious or severe infections were also very similar across all groups, as were the rates of laboratory abnormalities. No pattern of infection was observed in either study, but a slightly increased risk of infusion reactions was seen.[52] In BLISS-76, the rates of infusion reactions in the belimumab groups (1 mg/kg and 10 mg/kg) were 15.5% and 13.6%, respectively. The group that received belimumab at 10 mg/kg had a slightly increased risk of severe infusion reactions (1.1%), although rare, compared with the placebo group (0.4%).[53] In BLISS-52, the overall rates of infusion reactions in the treatment arms were comparable to those observed in the placebo arm. However, severe infusion reactions were slightly more common in both belimumab groups (1%) compared with the placebo group (<1%). No increase in the incidence or severity of AEs was observed in a 4-year continuation study of belimumab.[54]

Malignancy

No malignancies were reported in BLISS-52. In BLISS-76, malignancies occurred in 1.1% of patients in the belimumab arms, compared with 0.4% receiving placebo, although the authors believed this was consistent with previously reported malignancy rates in patients with SLE.

Suicidality

Because of the 3 completed and 4 attempted suicides, concern has been expressed about suicidality in patients participating in the belimumab studies. In BLISS-76, depression was reported more frequently in the belimumab groups (6%–7%) than in the placebo arm (4%).

Pregnancy

Only limited data exist for pregnancy in patients receiving belimumab. In BLISS-52, of 17 pregnancies with known outcomes, the rates of spontaneous abortion or stillbirth were similar in the treatment and placebo groups. In BLISS-76, no spontaneous abortions or stillbirths occurred in 5 pregnancies. Neither study reported any congenital abnormalities or postnatal complications.

OTHER DRUGS
Cyclosporine (Sandimmune, Neoral, Gengraf)

The most common AEs observed in patients receiving cyclosporine for autoimmune disease are

- Nephrotoxicity: this effect seems to be dose-dependent and can therefore be minimized by using the minimum effective dose (not to exceed 5 mg/kg/d), avoiding other potential nephrotoxins, and close monitoring of creatinine.[55]
- Hypertension
- Infection.

Thalidomide (Thalomid)

The most common AEs observed in patients receiving thalidomide for autoimmune disease are

- Peripheral neuropathy
- Drowsiness
- Constipation[56]
- Teratogenicity.

Adverse Events of Concern in SLE Patients Taking Commonly Prescribed Drugs
Nonsteroidal anti-inflammatory drugs

Nonsteroidal anti-inflammatory drugs (NSAIDs) are frequently prescribed for patients with SLE. Although NSAIDs should be used with caution because of common AEs, such as nephrotoxicity and peptic ulcer disease, patients with SLE seem to be at higher risk of aseptic meningitis while on NSAIDs compared with the general population. This AE occurs most frequently in patients taking ibuprofen.[57]

Glucocorticoids

Although osteonecrosis is a common AE experienced by patients treated with glucocorticoids, those with SLE are at increased risk for this complication. In a recent study of 337 patients taking glucocorticoids, the incidence of osteonecrosis was significantly higher in patients with SLE (37%) than in those without (21%). Risk factors include high initial corticosteroid doses[58] and SLE recurrence.[59] Several studies have observed no relationship to the duration of therapy or the total cumulative dose.

SUMMARY

Drugs used to treat SLE have a variety of toxicities. Physicians must familiarize themselves with all of the potential AEs and discuss the potential risks, along with possible alternatives, with patients to facilitate educated decision making.

REFERENCES

1. Firestein G, Budd R, Harris E Jr, et al. Kelley's textbook of rheumatology. 8th edition. Philadelphia: Elsevier Inc; 2009.

2. Cairoli E, Rebella M, Danese N, et al. Hydroxychloroquine reduces low-density lipoprotein cholesterol levels in systemic lupus erythematosus: a longitudinal evaluation of the lipid-lowering effect. Lupus, in press.

3. Ruiz-Irastorza G, Ramos-Casals M, Brito-Zeron P, et al. Clinical efficacy and side effects of antimalarials in systemic lupus erythematosus: a systematic review. Ann Rheum Dis 2010;69:20–8.

4. Alarcón GS, McGwin G, Bertoli AM, et al. Effect of hydroxychloroquine on the survival of patients with systemic lupus erythematosus: data from LUMINA, a multiethnic US cohort (LUMINA L). Ann Rheum Dis 2007;66:1168–72.

5. Shinjo SK, Bonfá E, Wojdyla D, et al. Antimalarial treatment may have a time-dependent effect on lupus survival: data from a multinational Latin American inception cohort. Arthritis Rheum 2010;62:855–62.

6. Aviña-Zubieta J, Galindo-Rodriguez G, Newman S, et al. Long-term effectiveness of antimalarial drugs in rheumatic diseases. Ann Rheum Dis 1998;57:582–7.

7. Leecharoen S, Wangkaew S, Louthrenoo W. Ocular side effects of chloroquine in patients with rheumatoid arthritis, systemic lupus erythematosus and scleroderma. J Med Assoc Thai 2007;90:52–8.

8. Levy GD, Munz SJ, Paschal J, et al. Incidence of hydroxychloroquine retinopathy in a large multicenter outpatient practice. Arthritis Rheum 1997;40:1482–6.

9. Wolfe F, Marmor MF. Rates and predictors of hydroxychloroquine retinal toxicity in patients with rheumatoid arthritis and systemic lupus erythematosus. Arthritis Care Res (Hoboken) 2010;62:775–84.

10. Marmor MF, Kellner U, Lai TY, et al. Revised recommendations on screening for chloroquine and hydroxychloroquine retinopathy. Ophthalmology 2011;118:415–22.

11. Hendrix JD, Greer KE. Cutaneous hyperpigmentation caused by systemic drugs. Int J Dermatol 1992;31:458–66.

12. Levantine A, Almeyda J. Drug induced changes in pigmentation. Br J Dermatol 1973;89:105–12.

13. Tuffanelli D, Abraham RK, Dubois EI. Pigmentation from antimalarial therapy. Arch Dermatol 1963;88:419.

14. Jover JA. Long-term use of antimalarial drugs in rheumatic diseases. Clin Exp Rheumatol 2012;30(3):380–7.

15. Makin AJ, Wendon J, Fitt S, et al. Fulminant hepatic failure secondary to hydroxychloroquine. Gut 1994;35:569–70.

16. Galvañ VG, Oltra MR, Rueda D, et al. Severe acute hepatitis related to hydroxychloroquine in a woman with mixed connective tissue disease. Clin Rheumatol 2007;26:971–2.

17. Weisholtz SJ, McBride PA, Murray HW, et al. Quinacrine-induced psychiatric disturbances. South Med J 1982;75(3):359–60.

18. Costedoat-Chalumeau N, Hulot JS, Amoura Z, et al. Cardiomyopathy related to antimalarial therapy with illustrative case report. Cardiology 2007;107(2):73–80.

19. Nord JE, Shah PK, Rinaldi RZ, et al. Hydroxychloroquine cardiotoxicity in systemic lupus erythematosus: a report of 2 cases and review of the literature. Semin Arthritis Rheum 2004;33:336–51.

20. Huskisson EC. Azathioprine. Clin Rheum Dis 1984;10(2):325–32.

21. Ford LT, Berg JD. Thiopurine S-methyltransferase (TPMT) assessment prior to starting thiopurine drug treatment; a pharmacogenomic test whose time has come. J Clin Pathol 2010;63:288–95.

22. Ragab AH, Gilkerson E, Myers M. The effect of 6-mercaptopurine and allopurinol on granulopoiesis. Cancer Res 1974;34(9):2246–9.

23. Johnson DH, Linde R, Hainsworth JD, et al. Effect of a luteinizing hormone releasing hormone agonist given during combination chemotherapy on posttherapy fertility in male patients with lymphoma: preliminary observations. Blood 1985;65(4):832–6.
24. Mok MY, Ng WL, Yuen MF, et al. Safety of disease modifying anti-rheumatic agents in rheumatoid arthritis patients with chronic viral hepatitis. Clin Exp Rheumatol 2000;18:363–8.
25. Østensen M, Khamashta M, Lockshin M, et al. Anti-inflammatory and immunosuppressive drugs and reproduction. Arthritis Res Ther 2006;8(3):209.
26. Radis CD, Kahl LE, Baker GL, et al. Effects of cyclophosphamide on the development of malignancy and on long-term survival of patients with rheumatoid arthritis. A 20-year followup study. Arthritis Rheum 1995;38(8):1120.
27. Bernatsky S, Joseph L, Boivin JF, et al. The relationship between cancer and medication exposures in systemic lupus erythaematosus: a case-cohort study. Ann Rheum Dis 2008;67(1):74–9.
28. Bernatsky S, Clarke AE, Suissa S. Hematologic malignant neoplasms after drug exposure in rheumatoid arthritis. Arch Intern Med 2008;168(4):378–81.
29. Mok CC, Ying KY, Ng WL, et al. Long-term outcome of diffuse proliferative lupus glomerulonephritis treated with cyclophosphamide. Am J Med 2006;119(4):355.
30. Appel GB, Contreras G, Dooley MA, et al. Mycophenolate mofetil versus cyclophosphamide for induction treatment of lupus nephritis. J Am Soc Nephrol 2009;20:1103–12.
31. Pryor BD, Bologna SG, Kahl LE. Risk factors for serious infection during treatment with cyclophosphamide and high-dose corticosteroids for systemic lupus erythematosus. Arthritis Rheum 1996;39(9):1475.
32. Uldall PR, Kerr DN, Tacchi D. Sterility and cyclophosphamide. Lancet 1972;1:693–4.
33. Austin HA 3rd, Klippel JH, Balow JE, et al. Therapy of lupus nephritis: controlled trial of prednisone and cytotoxic drugs. N Engl J Med 1986;314:614–9.
34. Houssiau FA, Vasconcelos C, D'Cruz D, et al. The 10-year follow-up data of the Euro-Lupus Nephritis Trial comparing low-dose and high dose intravenous cyclophosphamide. Ann Rheum Dis 2010;69:61–4.
35. Boumpas DT, Austin HA 3rd, Vaughan EM, et al. Risk for sustained amenorrhea in patients with systemic lupus erythematosus receiving intermittent pulse cyclophosphamide therapy. Ann Intern Med 1993;119(5):366–9.
36. Wang CL, Wang F, Bosco JJ. Ovarian failure in oral cyclophosphamide treatment for systemic lupus erythematosus. Lupus 1995;4(1):11.
37. Somers EC, Marder W, Christman GM, et al. Use of a gonadotropin-releasing hormone analog for protection against premature ovarian failure during cyclophosphamide therapy in women with severe lupus. Arthritis Rheum 2005;52(9):2761.
38. Blumenfeld Z, Shapiro D, Shteinberg M, et al. Preservation of fertility and ovarian function and minimizing gonadotoxicity in young women with systemic lupus erythematosus treated by chemotherapy. Lupus 2000;9(6):401.
39. Watson AR, Rance CP, Bain J. Long term effects of cyclophosphamide on testicular function. Br Med J (Clin Res Ed) 1985;291(6507):1457.
40. Waxman JH, Ahmed R, Smith D, et al. Failure to preserve fertility in patients with Hodgkin's disease. Cancer Chemother Pharmacol 1987;19(2):159.
41. Masala A, Faedda R, Alagna S, et al. Use of testosterone to prevent cyclophosphamide-induced azoospermia. Ann Intern Med 1997;126:292.
42. Cigni A, Faedda R, Atzeni MM, et al. Hormonal strategies for fertility preservation in patients receiving cyclophosphamide to treat glomerulonephritis: a nonrandomized trial and review of the literature. Am J Kidney Dis 2008;52(5):887–96.

43. Monach PA, Arnold LM, Merkel PA. Incidence and prevention of bladder toxicity from cyclophosphamide in the treatment of rheumatic diseases: a data-driven review. Arthritis Rheum 2010;62(1):9.

44. Riskalla MM, Somers EC, Fatica RA, et al. Tolerability of mycophenolate mofetil in patients with systemic lupus erythematosus. J Rheumatol 2003;30(7):1508.

45. Massari P, Duro-Garcia F, Girón E, et al. Safety assessment of the conversion from mycophenolate mofetil to enteric-coated mycophenolate sodium in stable renal transplant recipients. Transplant Proc 2005;37(2):916.

46. Dooley MA, Jayne D, Ginzler EM, et al. Mycophenolate versus azathioprine as maintenance therapy for lupus nephritis. N Engl J Med 2011;365:1886–95.

47. Merrill JT, Neuwelt CM, Wallace DJ, et al. Efficacy and safety of rituximab in moderately-to-severely active systemic lupus erythematosus. Arthritis Rheum 2010;62:222–33.

48. Rovin BH, Furie R, Latinis K. Efficacy and safety of rituximab in patients with active proliferative lupus nephritis: the Lupus Nephritis Assessment with Rituximab study. Arthritis Rheum 2012;64(4):1215–26.

49. Carson KR, Evens AM, Richey EA, et al. Progressive multifocal leukoencephalopathy after rituximab therapy in HIV-negative patients: a report of 57 cases from the Research on Adverse Drug Events and Reports project. Blood 2009; 113(20):4834.

50. Popa C, Leandro MJ, Cambridge G, et al. Repeated B lymphocyte depletion with rituximab in rheumatoid arthritis over 7 yrs. Rheumatology (Oxford) 2007;46(4): 626.

51. Keystone E, Fleischmann R, Emery P, et al. Safety and efficacy of additional courses of rituximab in patients with active rheumatoid arthritis: an open-label extension analysis. Arthritis Rheum 2007;56(12):3896.

52. Navarra SV, Guzmán RM, Gallacher AE, et al. Efficacy and safety of belimumab in patients with active systemic lupus erythematosus: a randomised, placebo-controlled, phase 3 trial. Lancet 2011;377:721–31.

53. Furie R, Petri M, Zamani O, et al. BLISS-76 Study Group. A phase III, randomized, placebo-controlled study of belimumab, a monoclonal antibody that inhibits B lymphocyte stimulator, in patients with systemic lupus erythematosus. Arthritis Rheum 2011;63:3918–30.

54. Merrill JT, Ginzler EM, Wallace DJ. Long-term safety profile of belimumab plus standard therapy in patients with systemic lupus erythematosus. Arthritis Rheum, in press.

55. Langford CA, Klippel JH, Balow JE, et al. Use of cytotoxic agents and cyclosporine in the treatment of autoimmune disease. Part 2: inflammatory bowel disease, systemic vasculitis, and therapeutic toxicity. Ann Intern Med 1998; 129(1):49–58.

56. Chang AY, Werth VP. Treatment of cutaneous lupus. Curr Rheumatol Rep 2011; 13(4):300–7.

57. Østensen M, Villiger PM. Nonsteroidal anti-inflammatory drugs in systemic lupus erythematosus. Lupus 2001;10(3):135–9.

58. Abeles M, Urman JD, Rothfield NF. Aseptic necrosis of bone in systemic lupus erythematosus. Relationship to corticosteroid therapy. Arch Intern Med 1978; 138(5):750.

59. Nakamura J, Ohtori S, Sakamoto M. Development of new osteonecrosis in systemic lupus erythematosus patients in association with long-term corticosteroid therapy after disease recurrence. Clin Exp Rheumatol 2010;28(1):13–8.

Index

Note: Page numbers of article titles are in **boldface** type.

Rheum Dis Clin N Am 38 (2012) 809–818
http://dx.doi.org/10.1016/S0889-857X(12)00092-0
0889-857X/12/$ – see front matter © 2012 Elsevier Inc. All rights reserved.

rheumatic.theclinics.com

United States Postal Service

Statement of Ownership, Management, and Circulation
(All Periodicals Publications Except Requester Publications)

1. Publication Title	2. Publication Number									3. Filing Date
Rheumatic Disease Clinics of North America	0	0	6	-	2	7	2			9/14/12

4. Issue Frequency	5. Number of Issues Published Annually	6. Annual Subscription Price
Feb, May, Aug, Nov	4	$305.00

7. Complete Mailing Address of Known Office of Publication (Not printer) (Street, city, county, state, and ZIP+4®)

Elsevier Inc.
360 Park Avenue South
New York, NY 10010-1710

Contact Person
Stephen Bushing
Telephone (Include area code)
215-239-3688

8. Complete Mailing Address of Headquarters or General Business Office of Publisher (Not printer)

Elsevier Inc., 360 Park Avenue South, New York, NY 10010-1710

9. Full Names and Complete Mailing Addresses of Publisher, Editor, and Managing Editor (Do not leave blank)

Publisher (Name and complete mailing address)

Kim Murphy, Elsevier, Inc., 1600 John F. Kennedy Blvd, Suite 1800, Philadelphia, PA 19103-2899

Editor (Name and complete mailing address)

Pamela Hetherington, Elsevier, Inc., 1600 John F. Kennedy Blvd, Suite 1800, Philadelphia, PA 19103-2899

Managing Editor (Name and complete mailing address)

Adrianne Brigido, Elsevier, Inc., 1600 John F. Kennedy Blvd. Suite 1800, Philadelphia, PA 19103-2899

10. Owner (Do not leave blank. If the publication is owned by a corporation, give the name and address of the corporation immediately followed by the names and addresses of all stockholders owning or holding 1 percent or more of the total amount of stock. If not owned by a corporation, give the names and addresses of the individual owners. If owned by a partnership or other unincorporated firm, give its name and address as well as those of each individual owner. If the publication is published by a nonprofit organization, give its name and address.)

Full Name	Complete Mailing Address
Wholly owned subsidiary of	1600 John F. Kennedy Blvd., Ste. 1800
Reed/Elsevier, US holdings	Philadelphia, PA 19103-2899

11. Known Bondholders, Mortgagees, and Other Security Holders Owning or Holding 1 Percent or More of Total Amount of Bonds, Mortgages, or Other Securities. If none, check box. ☐ None

Full Name	Complete Mailing Address
N/A	

12. Tax Status (For completion by nonprofit organizations authorized to mail at nonprofit rates) (Check one)
The purpose, function, and nonprofit status of this organization and the exempt status for federal income tax purposes:
☐ Has Not Changed During Preceding 12 Months
☐ Has Changed During Preceding 12 Months (Publisher must submit explanation of change with this statement)

PS Form 3526, September 2007 (Page 1 of 3 (Instructions Page 3)) PSN 7530-01-000-9931 PRIVACY NOTICE: See our Privacy policy in www.usps.com

---

13. Publication Title	14. Issue Date for Circulation Data Below
Rheumatic Disease Clinics of North America	May 2012

15. Extent and Nature of Circulation		Average No. Copies Each Issue During Preceding 12 Months	No. Copies of Single Issue Published Nearest to Filing Date
a. Total Number of Copies (Net press run)		1052	943
b. Paid Circulation (By Mail and Outside the Mail)	(1) Mailed Outside-County Paid Subscriptions Stated on PS Form 3541. (Include paid distribution above nominal rate, advertiser's proof copies, and exchange copies)	416	352
	(2) Mailed In-County Paid Subscriptions Stated on PS Form 3541 (Include paid distribution above nominal rate, advertiser's proof copies, and exchange copies)		
	(3) Paid Distribution Outside the Mails Including Sales Through Dealers and Carriers, Street Vendors, Counter Sales, and Other Paid Distribution Outside USPS®	269	233
	(4) Paid Distribution by Other Classes Mailed Through the USPS (e.g. First-Class Mail®)		
c. Total Paid Distribution (Sum of 15b (1), (2), (3), and (4))	►	685	585
d. Free or Nominal Rate Distribution (By Mail and Outside the Mail)	(1) Free or Nominal Rate Outside-County Copies Included on PS Form 3541	60	53
	(2) Free or Nominal Rate In-County Copies Included on PS Form 3541		
	(3) Free or Nominal Rate Copies Mailed at Other Classes Through the USPS (e.g. First-Class Mail)		
	(4) Free or Nominal Rate Distribution Outside the Mail (Carriers or other means)		
e. Total Free or Nominal Rate Distribution (Sum of 15d (1), (2), (3) and (4))	►	60	53
f. Total Distribution (Sum of 15c and 15e)	►	745	638
g. Copies not Distributed (See instructions to publishers #4 (page #3))	►	307	305
h. Total (Sum of 15f and g)	►	1052	943
i. Percent Paid (15c divided by 15f times 100)	►	91.95%	91.69%

16. Publication of Statement of Ownership

☐ If the publication is a general publication, publication of this statement is required. Will be printed in the November 2012 issue of this publication.   ☐ Publication not required

17. Signature and Title of Editor, Publisher, Business Manager, or Owner

Stephen R. Bushing   Stephen R. Bushing –Inventory Distribution Coordinator

Date
September 14, 2012

I certify that all information furnished on this form is true and complete. I understand that anyone who furnishes false or misleading information on this form or who omits material or information requested on the form may be subject to criminal sanctions (including fines and imprisonment) and/or civil sanctions (including civil penalties).

PS Form 3526, September 2007 (Page 2 of 3)

Moving?

Make sure your subscription moves with you!

To notify us of your new address, find your **Clinics Account Number** (located on your mailing label above your name), and contact customer service at:

Email: journalscustomerservice-usa@elsevier.com

800-654-2452 (subscribers in the U.S. & Canada)
314-447-8871 (subscribers outside of the U.S. & Canada)

Fax number: 314-447-8029

**Elsevier Health Sciences Division
Subscription Customer Service
3251 Riverport Lane
Maryland Heights, MO 63043**

*To ensure uninterrupted delivery of your subscription, please notify us at least 4 weeks in advance of move.

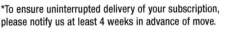

Printed and bound by CPI Group (UK) Ltd, Croydon, CR0 4YY

03/10/2024

01040440-0019